PRAISE FOR MOTHER

Modern life means so many new mothers struggle to find their footing alone, without the community support, wisdom—or even the bathroom break—that a village would have once provided. New moms often don't know how to make this transition easier. This book is a tremendous resource that offers something rare: a beautifully written mix of sage advice, personal and professional experience, and scientific evidence. It's a gift all moms should have.

—Tina Cassidy, author of *Birth: The Surprising History of How We Are Born*

Having a newborn is hard work, and while new mothers strive to provide the best possible care for their babies, it is also imperative that they take care of their own well-being. Finally there is a guidebook for new mothers about how to nourish not only their children, but also themselves. A must read!

—Dina DiMaggio, MD, pediatrician and coauthor of *The Pediatrician's Guide to Feeding Babies & Toddlers: Practical Answers to Your Questions on Nutrition, Starting Solids, Allergies, Picky Eating, and More*

Mother Matters is a sensitive, gentle, easy read for anyone who has a mother, is a mother, or wants to be a mother. Ms. Kurtz sprinkles interesting anecdotal examples and light research statistics into her down-to-earth, folksy style of writing, which makes this book an easy must-read for all!

—Fran Walfish, PsyD, Beverly Hills family and relationship psychotherapist and author of *The Self-Aware Parent*

Where has this book been hiding all these years—all these generations? With a remarkable ability to observe what is obvious but has remained unseen, Dayna Kurtz shares personal and professional insights in this thoughtful, practical, and cogent guide to mastering the challenges of motherhood. She speaks to the reader in an honest, authentic, and deeply personal voice, offering practical and scientifically validated interventions that can readily be implemented.

—Michael D. Zentman, PhD, Clinical psychologist and Associate Professor of Psychology and Director of the Postgraduate Program in Couple Therapy at Adelphi University

Drawing upon her experience as a seasoned psychotherapist and a dedicated mother, Dayna Kurtz's book, *Mother Matters*, is deeply compassionate, yet imminently practical, and an essential addition to anyone seeking a more profound, rich, and evocative understanding of motherhood.

—Sebastian Zimmermann, MD, psychiatrist and author of *Fifty Shrinks*

Mother Matters is a warm, witty, and practical guide to helping new mothers navigate the often breathtaking, but sometimes difficult and rarely perfect, transition into motherhood. Bolstered by the latest findings in scientific research and her own training as a clinical social worker and certified pre- and postnatal fitness trainer, author Dayna Kurtz offers practical "how-to" advice, illustrative real-life vignettes, and her own poignant reflections on the vicissitudes of motherhood. Kurtz's writing style is clear, pragmatic, and to the point. Recognizing the societal pressures women face to "do it all" and to do it flawlessly, especially when it comes to motherhood, Kurtz emphasizes the importance of making room for imperfection and of caring for mother as well as baby. This book will be invaluable to new moms and to those who love them.

—Karen Starr, PsyD, clinical psychologist and psychoanalyst

Today's mother gets pulled in so many directions, it's no wonder so many put their own self-care on the back burner. *Mother Matters* guides you, the ever-sacrificing mom, through the essential steps of keeping yourself healthy, strong, and sane through the joyful madness we call motherhood.

—Dan DeFigio, founder of BeatingSugarAddiction.com and author of *Beating Sugar Addiction for Dummies*

MOTHER MATTERS

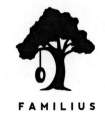

FAMILIUS

Published by Familius LLC, www.familius.com

Familius books are available at special discounts for bulk purchases, whether for sales promotions or for family or corporate use. For more information, contact Familius Sales at 559-876-2170 or email orders@familius.com.

Library of Congress Catalog-in-Publication Data
2017962272

Print ISBN 9781945547782
Ebook ISBN 9781641700290

Printed in the United States of America

Edited by Michele Robbins
Cover design by David Miles
Book design by Brooke Jorden and Caroline Larsen

10 9 8 7 6 5 4 3 2 1

First Edition

MOTHER MATTERS

A HOLISTIC GUIDE TO BEING A HAPPY, HEALTHY MOM

DAYNA M. KURTZ, LMSW, CPT

My eight-year-old son, Asher, was the first to spread the news when I signed my book contract. He told our doorman, strangers on the elevator, his teachers, and anyone else who happened to cross his path. His enthusiasm for my work did not rival my own, it surpassed it. Indeed, his enthusiasm for life is a wonder to behold; a source of inspiration and a worthy aspiration. Asher's influence on me is unparalleled, as is that of all children, I imagine, on their parents.

Asher, being your mother informs the way I move through the world and the mark I hope to leave on it. Thank you for giving me the gift of motherhood, my gorgeous boy. I love you.

TABLE OF CONTENTS

INTRODUCTION

I was primed to be a good mom. As a social worker trained in counseling others, I spent many years in my own therapy gaining deeper insight into myself. A more refined self-awareness served me well in navigating a privileged life—selecting a career to which I was well suited, choosing a loving partner, and making a mindful decision to become a parent. That last choice, made with thoughtful and careful reflection, was bolstered by the confidence of knowing I was in a place with every resource at my disposal: family help, a supportive husband, financial stability, health, and the desire for a child. I was indeed blessed and believed I was prepared to become a successful mama. To my surprise, my entry into motherhood was something of a *failure to thrive*. This term usually refers to infants whose growth is stunted by a lack of nourishment; as a new mom, I suffered from not knowing how to feed myself. In hindsight, it was this critical resource—a reliable, protective guide to transport me smoothly across the bridge into the mother world—that was missing. And it would have made a huge difference in coping with the cultural mandate to breastfeed successfully, lose the baby weight rapidly, sleep-train effectively, and (co)parent seamlessly. Knowing how to care for the new mother in me was far more important (I now know) than all the self-knowledge and all the professional experience I had in helping others. Without it, my transition to maternal life was a messy, painful journey. Every emotional, physical, and spiritual part of my being was poured into child-rearing, leaving a depleted shell of the woman I had worked so hard to know well. By all accounts my baby was, thankfully, healthy and seemingly happy. Did that make me a good mom? If so, if this was what good mothering required, I didn't know how I would survive it. Starved of soul-food, my pre-parent self was eclipsed by a hostile, short-tempered, unrecognizable being.

This became strikingly apparent when my son reached one month old. Seated on a slowly deflating exercise ball with my baby cradled in my arms, I had just entered into the second hour of a slow, rhythmic bounce, trying unsuccessfully to woo him to sleep. And then my husband called.

"Hi Sweetie, I just left the office."

"Yes. And?"

"I'm on my way home. I just wanted to call."

"Okay. So?"

"Did you see the moon? It's huge and full. Just beautiful."

"The moon? Did I see the moon?! No! I didn't see the moon! I didn't see the moon because I've been trying to get our child to sleep for the last hour by bouncing my butt off!"

So much for romance.

Donald Winnicott, noted British pediatrician and psychoanalyst, researched and wrote extensively about the mother-infant relationship. He affirmed what we all know intellectually: a perfect mother does not exist. "Perfection," he stated, "belongs to machines" (Winnicott 1971, 163). Winnicott made a case for the fundamental importance of a mother who is imperfect—who is merely "good enough." The "good enough" mother is one who strives to meet most of her child's needs, but not all (1953, 89–97). As baby grows, mother gradually allows her to develop her own capabilities, providing opportunities to learn to overcome challenges. In so doing, the hope is she will become a secure, independent person in her own right (1953, 94).

Even if it were possible, striving for maternal perfection would be futile, doing a disservice to both a mother and her child. And frankly, as I discovered, simply striving to be "good enough," is hard enough. Contemporary psychoanalyst and feminist Jessica Benjamin takes Winnicott's notion one step further. In not meeting her child's every need, the "good enough" mother also allows a chance for her child to develop a fundamental understanding—that her mother is a separate person. Learning to recognize mother as an individual can help the child develop a "shared understanding"—the basis of empathy—and is essential in being able to connect and build stable relationships (Benjamin 1995, 193). As a new mother, every day presents innumerable moments to grow into the parent one hopes to be. With each of these moments also comes the challenge of finding a balance between the needs of the child and the needs of her mother.

Though the birth of a baby happens in a matter of hours, the birth of a mother is an ongoing, evolutionary process. As a baby explores the new world around her, a mother is similarly exploring and growing into her new role. How do you reconcile the woman you once were with the mother you are becoming? How can you be not only good enough, but also thrive? How can you find time to gaze at the beauty of a full moon? Figuring out how to do these things—how to feed not only my child but also myself—changed my life for the better. Learning how to do these things will change your life for the better, too. There is no magic formula here, no hocus-pocus. There is simply science; solid research of what has worked for countless mothers and an irrefutable argument that every mother deserves access to it. Making the work of mothering easier is a matter of having the right tools for the job. *Mother Matters* is the comprehensive tool kit.

MOTHERCARE, REALIZED

Not only is the work of mothering impossible to quantify, but the act of becoming a mother is in and of itself an extraordinary feat of perseverance, strength, and endurance. And, I realized, it necessitates an intelligently designed, comprehensive, custom-tailored, and practical support system. Thus began my mission: to research, study, and make accessible a wide array of strategies for self-care that can help make the transition to motherhood easier and more enjoyable.

Deeply familiar with the benefits of talk-therapy as a provider and a patient, this support was a comfortable and effective place to begin my search. Given my personal experience, I also knew it was not enough. I needed much more. Where to look? The answer, surprisingly, was right outside my door—literally. Every November, the New York City Marathon runs up First Avenue in Manhattan. Every year I would venture outside and watch as tens of thousands of people would run together toward the same finish line. Every year I would cry—the kind of tears that flow from a source deep within the soul. Part of what so touched me about the marathon was the juxtaposition of its insurmountability and its accessibility. Nearly every shape and size runner was represented—every color, young and old. As one who grew up chubby and athletically challenged, I watched with awe and a curious yearning about the possibility of fitting in with this pack. Which is why, I know now, when my husband declared, "You should run it," I said, "Yes." It made no sense. But the soul that shed those tears knew I had to do it. My marathon training, coinciding with my son's growth from one to two years, had a marked effect on my happiness. Returning from a run, I observed in myself a new sense of calm and a more patient, enthusiastic approach in relating to my child. The research on exercise as a natural mood booster is well-documented. But having never before experienced it myself, I wondered about the use of exercise at this particular juncture in a woman's life. How great an impact could it be on a new mother's overall healing and well-being? I returned to school to better understand exercise science and became a certified pre- and postnatal fitness trainer. From there, I continued to seek out and research better and lesser known tools that I hypothesized might be of benefit to new moms—acupressure, expressive-arts therapy, and diet—to name just a few.

This book is the culmination of that effort. *Mother Matters* serves as a reliable, informative, and non-judgmental guide for each new mother, helping you assess where you might benefit the most from assistance, providing you with concrete tools, and offering you resources for when additional help may be useful. It may be read from cover-to-cover for a well-stocked tool kit of helpful techniques or used as a reference guide by perusing chapters of particular interest; those are likely to be the ones that resonate and will be most useful. The vignettes provided throughout the book illustrate how mothers use these tools to ease the maternal transition. To protect their privacy, all names and identifying information of the individuals' stories presented herein have been changed. The vignettes presented are largely composites drawn from mothers with whom I have worked in clinical practice.

This information is not intended as a substitute for medical advice. Readers should consult their doctors with specific questions pertaining to their own health. If you are experiencing profound sadness or irritability, or have lost interest in activities you once enjoyed, please reach out to your healthcare provider immediately. If you are having disturbing thoughts of harming yourself or your baby, call 911.

Wherever you are on the spectrum, whether trying to conceive, pregnant, with a newborn at home, or waiting for a call from the adoption agency, someone else is feeling exactly as you do now. Becoming a mother, though deeply personal, is also an experience shared by countless women around the world. Whether anxious or scared, exhausted or overwhelmed, elated, confounded, unsure, or all of these at once, many others are feeling just the same. Welcome to motherhood. It is an honor to be with you.

CHILDCARE. ELDERCARE. MOTHERCARE?

WHAT'S *MOTHERCARE?*

The care that women receive as they grapple with the multiple transitions of postpartum is at best highly fragmented and at worst close to nonexistent relative to their needs during this time.

—Tekoa L. King, Midwife

I n hospitals, birthing centers, and homes, nearly four million babies are born in America every year according to the Center for Disease Control (2015). As these newborns enter the world, millions of quieter births are taking place, too. Though not documented on birth certificates or recorded by the government, these emerging identities are just as beautiful, just as compelling and worthy of attention. Every year, millions of mothers are born.

Becoming a mother is a complex transition, layered with profound and intense emotion. Among the biggest of life's privileges, motherhood affords an opportunity to experience unparalleled love and incomparable joy. And, like many heightened privileges, the entrée to motherhood also brings enormous responsibility, peppered with feelings of anxiety, guilt, anger, and fear.

Most jobs offer some sort of training—an orientation, a chance to shadow an experienced employee, an instruction manual. Motherhood, often described as the hardest job there is, offers none of these. New mothers are led to believe *maternal instinct* and *mother's intuition* are the natural tendencies that will help them to gracefully embrace this new role. But how can instinct and intuition help moms navigate the agony of sleep deprivation, the mechanics of breastfeeding (if they so choose), the social isolation, the career negotiation, the management of co-parenting or single-parenting, and the multitude of other trials that leave mothers understandably overwhelmed—especially in the beginning? Maternal instinct and intuition are meant to help mothers care for their *babies*. They are valuable guides, but they are not enough. New mothers need to know how to care for *themselves*. They need something more than intuition and instinct. They need an arsenal of reliable supports.

Having a baby is so commonplace, so natural. After all, it happens all day, every day, up to four million times in a year! But nature doesn't always mean sunny skies and starry nights. Sometimes it means pounding hail and dust storms, too. The early years of motherhood offer the full spectrum of natural weather. By learning to take care of the mother-self, one can greatly improve the forecast for herself, her baby, and her family. Few people dispute

New mothers need something more than intuition and instinct. They need an arsenal of reliable supports.

that tending to the body, mind, and spirit are essential to living a healthy and happy life. And yet, during one of the most complex, stressful, and overwhelming of life's transitions, new moms often

This is not a book about how to raise a happy, healthy child. This is a book about how to raise a happy, healthy mother.

get short shrift. Doesn't that seem backward? Shouldn't mothers be getting *more* support at this critical life-stage? Shouldn't someone teach them, for example, that acupressure can actually bolster milk production and lower levels of the stress hormone cortisol? Wouldn't it be helpful for them to be shown a simple coloring exercise that improves feelings of productivity and enables mother-infant bonding? What if every new mother were taught which foods can directly impact physical healing from labor and delivery and enhance emotional health? These ideas are not the stuff of daydreams. They are facts steeped in science. Every mother should have access to them.

This is not a book about how to raise a happy, healthy child. There are plenty of those. This is a book about how to raise a happy, healthy mother. That's a subject that needs to be talked about more.

MOTHERDOM OR MARTYRDOM?

A frightening trend has infiltrated motherhood. The expectations on mothers have become boundless. If mothering was the hardest job in the world before, it has become harder still. The pressures on today's moms are sky-high, while the resources afforded them are few and far between. In overt and subtle ways, the message being sent to us is that the maternal experience does not matter, that to be a good mother means to be a good martyr. Over and over again, everywhere we turn, moms are getting the message. And we are answering the call. Unfortunately, the results have devastating implications for ourselves, for our babies, and for our families.

POSTPARTUM CHECKUP OR CHECKOUT?: LIZ'S STORY

Six weeks after giving birth, I sat in a blue paper gown in a generic exam room at my ob-gyn's office, awaiting my postnatal checkup. I was still tremendously sore from the episiotomy I endured to prevent what my doctor told me would have been traumatic tearing. I remember cringing when I thought about what my doctor might see down there. My thought was interrupted by my baby, Liam's, shriek, waking from what felt like only a momentary nap, demanding to be fed. I could feel my cheeks flush—a feeling that had become familiar in recent days. "Do I have time to nurse him before the doctor comes in?" I worried. "What if I start and have to stop? What will the doctor think of me? And don't forget to ask him about the pain around my incision scar. Why does it still hurt so much?" The thoughts flitted in and out of my mind like gnats swarming under a porch light. A few moments later, Dr. Silver came in.

"There's that gorgeous boy," he said, "and how's the new mom?"

"I'm okay," I said, forcing a half-smile. "Um, tired."

"Of course, you are," my doctor replied, in a way that felt dismissive. "You're a new mother!"

He examined me, told me I was "cleared for sex," and asked if I wanted to discuss birth control options. The appointment was so swift, and he seemed like he was in such a rush, I didn't have an opportunity to ask about anything pertaining to my well-being. The floodgates opened before I could even get my clothes on. I realized I would wind up leaving the office still wondering when, or if, I might feel normal again.

Not long after that first postpartum checkup, many moms are in the position of either needing to or choosing whether to return to work outside the home. Monique is one of the nearly 70 percent of women with children under eighteen who are either employed or seeking employment, according to the 2015 Bureau of Labor Statistics report. Like most new mothers, Monique found herself spending more hands-on time child-rearing, as well as more time in the workplace, than her mother and grandmother had done before her. Without access to paid maternity leave for any given amount of time, Monique was in the all-too-familiar position of needing to return to work before she felt ready.

WORK AND NO PAY MAKES A REAL MESS OF THINGS: MONIQUE'S STORY

I wasn't sure I really wanted to return to work at all. I loved the intellectual stimulation and my work friends, but Daryl was still so tiny. I remember wishing, "If I just had a few more months, maybe this would all be easier—it would be better for all of us." But I had already used up three months unpaid family leave time from my company and an additional month of saved vacation time. I carried the health insurance. There was no choice involved. Those first months back were pretty awful. My boss called me into her office at one point to review the 'sub-par' quality of my performance on a number of recent projects. Total humiliation. I remember thinking, "Now I suck at both my jobs—motherhood and sales." By the time I would get home at night, my exhaustion and frustration set me and my husband, Jamal, up for regular screaming matches. We always used to communicate so well, but suddenly it felt as though we couldn't discuss anything—from daycare to dishes—without biting the other's head off. I actually began to wonder if our marriage would ever be happy again, and even if it would survive our having had a baby!

If Monique had become a mother during her grandmother's time, she may well have had an entirely different experience. In 1940, a generation of moms were forced into factories to do the work of their husbands who were at war overseas. The Lanham Act established a collective of government-run childcare centers serving thousands of children across all income levels. The centers of the early '40s were forward-thinking, smartly designed, and well-equipped to serve the needs of even today's moms. Apart from a play space for children, the day cares also consisted of the following amenities: a tailor (because what mother of young children has time to hem a skirt?), a supermarket (with employees who would complete grocery shopping based on mom's list and have it ready and waiting at pick-up time), and a medical clinic (staffed by professional healthcare workers who could provide vaccinations and other routine health maintenance).

These resources were in addition to the infirmary, where sons and daughters could be left in able-bodied hands on sick days, so moms would not run the risk of being fired for needing to stay home. Finally, the pièce de résistance, a take-out counter replete with chicken dinners and all the fixings. All a mom had to do was bring it home and heat it up. The Lanham Act was put to bed after the war ended and men returned stateside. But the precedent for federally funded, equal-access childcare in America remains. Imagine how Monique's experience of early mothering might be different if her day care situation was covered—and so was dinner?

Ashley lives in Melbourne, Australia. When she brought her daughter, Kat, home from the hospital, she planned on following the guidelines issued by the Australian National Health and Medical Research Council, that babies should be exclusively breastfed for six months. Kat's pediatrician endorsed this belief, pointing out that "breast is best" for Kat's health and development.

Ashley's "natural" experience of breastfeeding turned out to be dark and stormy, not to mention painful.

IF *BREAST IS BEST*, WHY IS BREASTFEEDING SO HARD?: ASHLEY'S STORY

The ache in my nipples was almost intolerable. I pumped—it seemed constantly—but I was barely able to get more than an ounce or two at a sitting. I remember thinking that nursing was the most natural thing in the world, and I couldn't understand why I was struggling so much. "Bad mother," I would tell myself. Everyone around me said "breast is best," so I figured I had to keep at it. When Kat was four weeks old, the pain in my left breast was so overwhelming I nearly passed out. My husband insisted I see the doctor. Turns out I had developed severe mastitis—a common infection. The abscess I developed had to be surgically drained, and I was unable to care for my baby at all during that time. My mom had to take time off work—unpaid, of course—to care for both me and my baby girl. I knew she was not in a financial position to do it and that stressed both of us out.

Dr. Julie Smith of the Australian Center for Economic Research on Health recently investigated the logistics of the breastfeeding recommendation, which is shared by the American Academy of Pediatrics. She found, on average, a nursing mother who follows the guideline needs to spend about eighteen hours a week on newborn feeding alone. By contrast, mothers who use solids or formula spend about 6.6 fewer hours on feeding (Smith and Forrester 2013, 3–4). Ashley was an adoring, competent, and dedicated new mom, but even Wonder Woman (Wonder Mother?!) would have struggled to make that work.

THE MISTAKES OF BEING MOTHERCARE-LESS

Liz, Monique, and Ashley are loving, smart, all-around terrific mothers. They were doing everything right in a system that is all-too wrong. Mothers are expected to make magic happen without being given any tricks to keep up their sleeves. They are expected to manage the extraordinary task of caring for their babies while keeping up at the office and steadying the day-to-day life in-between. And, as is clear from the cases of these three moms and countless others, they are meant to do it without accessible, reliable, tangible help. The result is a generation of mothers who have been completely depleted of their resources. They are overwhelmed and under-well, and the results are tragic.

How many mothers have been in Liz's position? How many mothers have been at a postpartum checkup, a pediatrician visit, or even at a new moms' group and felt that the only cries being heard were the ones of their babies? When women are not afforded opportunities to share their candid experiences of early mothering in a supportive, non-judgmental way, everyone suffers. Mothers suffer. Their babies suffer too.

Feelings are like babies themselves. They need to be born and delivered out into the world. When people, mothers or not, are unable to give voice to how they feel, uncomfortable emotions fester and are turned inward. These pent-up feelings can metastasize into depression and anxiety. Beyond the maternal anguish, a large body of research points to the effects this depression has on babies, including the risk of stunted growth to their social, emotional, and cognitive development.

How many mothers have found themselves in Monique's dilemma? How many mothers have been forced to return to work before they felt ready to do so or in spite of their preference to remain at home. In 2011, the non-profit NGO Human Rights Watch published *Failing its Families: Lack of Paid Leave and Work-Family Supports in the US*. The report highlighted interviews with parents who needed to return to work before they

When women are not afforded opportunities to share their candid experiences of early mothering in a supportive, non-judgmental way, everyone suffers. Mothers suffer. Their babies suffer too.

might otherwise have done so due to minimal or no paid leave following the birth or adoption of a baby. Mothers echoed the ill effects of no paid family leave, including: having to miss vaccinations or appointments, stopping breastfeeding before they were ready, and feeling depressed as a result of having to be at work.

How many mothers, like Ashley, have questioned the state of their marriages following the birth of a baby? A study published in the *Journal of Personality and Social Psychology* followed 218 heterosexual couples over the first eight years of their marriage. Mothers and fathers reported a sharp decrease in relationship functionality following the birth of a first baby. This decrease in functionality affected couples over the course of the eight-year study. Couples without children also reported some decline in how well their marriages were working, but these declines happened much more slowly and gradually. Researchers concluded that the sudden changes observed in the new parents were likely the result of the birth of a child (Doss, Rhoades, Stanley, and Markman 2009, 601–619). One might wonder: Was it the birth of the child itself, the state of motherhood today, or the interplay between the two?

MOTHERCARE BEGINS NOW

Liz, Monique, and Ashley deserve to be mothering in a better environment. Most mothers today deserve to be mothering in a better environment. The system needs a shift. Ideally, the demands on mothers need to be relaxed and the supports given to them need to be enhanced. But what do mothers do in the meantime? What do they do to break the cycle of martyrdom and reclaim the pleasure, the privilege, of motherhood? They start by taking care of themselves. Mother*hood* is about taking care of a baby. Mother*care* is about taking care of mom. Becoming a mother requires doing *both*. One should not, cannot, exist without the other.

When a woman has a child the focus is on her baby. This is as it should be. But when a woman becomes a mother, focus, attention, and care can and should expand to celebrate the multiple births taking place, not only that of a baby, but also of a mother. Just as an infant is thrust into a curious world, one which inundates the senses, his mother is similarly entering an unknown universe, rich in new, challenging experiences and overwhelming emotion. Like her baby, a mother also needs to be held and cradled.

The tools described in the coming chapters are simple to understand, easy to use, cost-effective, and do not require a big time commitment. They can be used right now, today, to make the work of motherhood easier by helping you learn how to take better, move loving care of yourself.

When a woman becomes a mother, focus, attention, and care can and should expand to celebrate the multiple births taking place, not only that of a baby, but also of a mother.

It bears repeating: this is not a book about how to raise a happy, healthy child. It is a book about how to raise a happy, healthy mother. The cliché that taking care of yourself will make you better able to care for your baby is true. A better nourished mother will make for a better nourished baby. If holding on to this truth is what you need to begin using the resources ahead, by all means, do so. Please bear in mind, too, that the mandate for mothercare recognizes the value of feeling well as a right not just of every mom, but of every human being. And moms are special human beings indeed. Congratulations! The path to happier, healthier motherhood begins now.

ACUPUNCTURE & ACUPRESSURE

THE BENEFITS OF PINS & NEEDLES

Acupuncture is a jab well done.

—Unknown

I n Western culture, needles are often associated with shots, illicit drug use, and body piercing. But in the Far East, it's a far different story. In this part of the world, needles have been connected with a therapeutic method of healing for centuries. Acupuncture is the ancient practice of using strategically placed, paper-thin needles just below the skin to stimulate the flow of *Qi* (chee). Licensed acupuncturist and researcher Stephen

Birch writes that the concept of Qi dates back as early as 150–400 BCE and describes it as a kind of life energy or force that flows through us (2015, 59). In Traditional Chinese Medicine (TCM), when the flow of Qi is blocked, the result can be ill health. Qi that is prevented from moving fluidly can manifest in the form of more minor ailments, like head or backaches, to more serious diseases, like cancer. According to TCM, acupuncture aims to unblock the flow of Qi, thereby enabling healing and well-being.

Meridians are particular regions through which Qi—the life energy—as well as blood and other bodily fluids, are believed to travel. Meridian maps organize the body into these different sections, which help determine needle placement and course of treatment. While not actually visible the way bones and organs are, the twelve meridians that guide acupuncture treatment are an integral part of the process, informing practitioners about what may be happening inside the body.

News reports point out that recent years have seen an uptick in the use of acupuncture as both a primary and complementary intervention in Western medicine (Samadi 2012). While TCM understands acupuncture's effectiveness through the unblocking of Qi, Western medicine offers a different explanation: studies demonstrate measurable changes in body chemistry as a result of the technique. This contributes to the popular consensus in the West that acupuncture's effectiveness is a product of the way it stimulates the nervous system.

While women transition into the postpartum period, acupuncture can be employed as an effective support in handling the frequent challenges that arise. Pain relief following a Caesarean section and stimulation of milk production are both instances in which acupuncture has been used with great success (Zhao and Guo 2006, 29–30). Women who suffer from headaches or backaches in the postnatal period may find that acupuncture can be an especially helpful tool in limiting discomfort and maintaining health.

MANAGING UTERINE PAIN: BELLA'S STORY

I've had bad PMS almost as long as I've been getting my period. My cramps would get so intense at times that I would have to stay home from school or work. My mood? Forget it. I was impossible to be around. I was irritable and would cry at the drop of a hat. When I began taking a birth control pill, that helped a little. My periods were lighter and the cramping was more manageable. I was still pretty moody though, and I just didn't feel like myself for those five days out of the month. When I went off the pill to try and get pregnant I was afraid about how I would manage the PMS if I didn't conceive right away. I'm not a fan of needles, but I asked my ob-gyn about acupuncture and she agreed it might help with the symptoms. She gave me the name of a licensed acupuncturist and I scheduled my first appointment. I was really nervous, but the treatment itself was actually pretty relaxing—no pain whatsoever where the needles were concerned. When I got my period the fourth month after coming off the pill, I noticed my cramps were not as intense as usual and my moods felt more stable. I continued to see my acupuncturist weekly throughout my pregnancy!

Women who suffer from headaches or backaches in the postnatal period may find that acupuncture can be an especially helpful tool in limiting discomfort and maintaining health.

For those who can't get past the needle factor or do not have easy access to a licensed acupuncturist, acu*pressure* is a smart alternative. Developed five thousand years ago, acupressure is essentially a form of massage that works along the same Eastern and Western principles, either by removing blocks to the flow of

Developed five thousand years ago, acupressure is essentially a form of massage that works along the same Eastern and Western principles, either by removing blocks to the flow of Qi or by positively affecting the nervous system.

Qi or by positively affecting the nervous system. Instead of using specialized needles, however, the practitioner uses fingers to apply pressure to particular points on the body.

One scientific theory that explains how acupressure may be effective suggests that the points on the body where pressure is applied are actually physiologically distinct from other locations on the body. These specific regions, known as acupoints or Tsubos, are believed to have a greater number of neuroreceptors. Neuroreceptors receive input from neurotransmitters, like dopamine, which control the *pleasure center* in the brain. The communication between the neurotransmitter and its receptor profoundly impacts the chemical reactions of a cell. Acupressure may work by interrupting or halting pain or other impulses produced at these highly sensitive sites (Jimenez 1995, 7–10).

In coping with the realities of postpartum life, acupressure can be a really effective *hands-on* (sorry—couldn't resist) strategy. This treatment can help with healing after childbirth, promoting lactation, and lessening the debilitating effects of sleep deprivation, stress, and baby blues.

EASING THE PAIN POST C-SECTION: BETHANY'S STORY

After ten hours of labor that didn't progress, my obstetrician and I decided that I should have a C-section. To my great relief, Kayla was born healthy and happy. After her birth, though, I was kind of a mess. The incision was so sore I could barely move. For the first couple of weeks back at home, I had to sleep on the couch because the stairs up to the bedroom were just too difficult to climb.

I was concerned about using anything stronger than a heating pad since I was nursing. Acupressure was a lifesaver. My husband had learned some techniques during a birthing class we took together. I had actually forgotten about it until he suggested trying a few pressure points. I don't know whether it was his healing touch or the actual acupressure itself, but the pain around the incision site started to go away pretty quickly. Kayla is three now, and I still ask Tom to use acupressure on me when I have a headache or trouble sleeping. More often than not, it does the trick!

Recently, a group of women recovering from C-sections received a series of Auricular (ear) acupressure treatments, twice daily in the week directly following birth. At five days postpartum, this group was found to have lower levels of the stress hormone cortisol, lower heart rates, and lower levels of anxiety and fatigue than their peers who did not receive treatment (Kuy, Tsai, Tzeng, and Chen 2016, 17–26).

A different group of mothers experienced the benefits of acupressure as a means of managing hypogalactica, insufficient or below average milk production. Mothers ranging from ten days to six months postpartum were given basic instruction on how and where to apply pressure and administered the technique on themselves. Milk production was measured using an electric breast pump at two and four weeks following the introduction of the acupressure treatment. The average volume of milk collected increased significantly (Esfahani et al. 2015, 7–11).

Working with a licensed acupuncturist or a massage therapist schooled in acupressure can be a good way to become acquainted with how the treatment works. If your time and budget allow, even one session with a professional can help you identify points on the body and how much pressure to use. This can greatly enhance the ability for self-practice afterward. Many practitioners will provide in-home treatment, and some accept insurance.

ACUPRESSURE: SELF-PRACTICE FOR MOMS

While acupuncture should not be self-administered (I don't know many people inclined to take a needle to themselves anyhow), acupressure can be easily practiced by almost anyone at any time. Before doing so, it is important to understand some very basic facts about application, as well as where to locate the specific pressure points on the body.

To begin, find a quiet, relaxing space and sit comfortably. Close your eyes and bring attention to your breath. Breathing should be easy, with effortless inhalations and exhalations. Starting from a place of greater relaxation can add to the value of the exercise. Consider the intention for your practice; is it stress relief? Rebuilding strength after labor? Promoting lactation? Perhaps all of the above. Knowing which acupressure points to focus on can help you to derive greater benefit, especially when your time is so limited. In terms of the amount of pressure to use, an achy sensation should occur around the acupoint site, but it should not feel painful. One indication that may be used to assess pressure is to notice your fingernail. Press hard enough on the point using the pad of your thumb or finger so that the skin underneath the nail begins to turn white. When first beginning to practice the technique, choose a point where the thumb or finger may be easily observed, until the right amount of pressure becomes second nature. While there is no disadvantage to doing too much acupressure, aiming to treat points twice a day is plenty. And of course, there will be many days when finding time for even one treatment will be a worthy accomplishment.

Ashley Flores, licensed acupuncturist and owner of Four Flowers Wellness in Chicago, works with many postpartum clients. She offers the following suggestions for the self-guided practices outlined below.

PERICARDIUMS 5, 6, AND 7

Why to do it: Applying pressure to the pericardium points can be helpful in regaining strength and recovering from labor. In Eastern terminology, attending to these acupressure points can stimulate blood flow, aid in building Qi, and support general wellness. They can help new mothers to feel calmer, more grounded, and less anxious. Practitioners will sometimes treat these points by way of helping clients to *turn off* worry and make them better able to transition from one task to the next. Applying acupressure to the Pericardiums 5, 6, and 7 can be especially useful before going to sleep as a means of moving away from wakefulness and toward rest.

How to do it: Pericardiums 5, 6, and 7 are found at the inside of the wrist. To find them, look at the inside of your wrist and locate the two tendons in the center. (If they are not visible at first, flex the wrist back and forth until they are either seen or can be felt with your index finger.) Take the thumb of your opposite hand and place it two thumb-widths up from your wrist crease, toward the elbow. Place your thumb parallel to the wrist and begin to massage in a circular motion. Gentle pressure should be applied, enough to feel a bit of an ache on the spot but not pain. It does not matter which wrist you chose to treat first, but do massage both sides for about thirty seconds to a minute each.

LIVER 5, WORM HOLE

Why to do it: So named because of the depression in the bone that resembles where the invertebrate might make his home, the Liver 5 point is the one to target to improve any vaginal inflammation or urinary issues, or if there was any tearing or cutting around the perineum during labor.

How to do it: About midway between the knee and ankle on the inside of the leg along the bone there is a series of slight depressions or tender spots. Using your thumb, apply pressure on the spot until a mild soreness or achy feeling develops. Some women will experience a kind of warmth radiating from the point or a sense of connectedness with the area. The point may begin to feel softer or there may be a sense that the depression is beginning to fill in some way. Spend about thirty seconds to a minute on each side.

INNER YIN

Why to do it: Toward the end of pregnancy many moms are all-too-familiar with the discomfort of fatigue and heaviness in their legs. In the weeks and months postpartum, your legs may find relief with a little attention paid to the *Inner Yin.* These points can enable healthy circulation, bringing blood from the legs back to the rest of the body, and may ease swelling in the lower extremities. The Inner Yin points are also treated in cases of lower abdominal pain and discomfort in the pubic area. For those who may have had an IV during labor and delivery, these points can help in the reduction of postpartum swelling. Finally, a little attention to the Inner Yin can provide some much-needed relief to the shoulder, neck, and spine muscles, often in desperate need of some TLC after all that baby-carrying!

How to do it: Sit on the floor butterfly style with the soles of your feet facing each other. Between the knee and the crease by the pubic area, right in the middle of the inner thigh, sit the Inner Yin points. Using your right elbow, begin by gently pressing down on the inside of your right thigh, above (but NOT on) the knee. Continue this application of pressure while working up toward the pubic area. Take about thirty seconds to complete one pass and then repeat four or five times, being sure to do both legs one at a time. Those who prefer not to use an elbow may use a foam roller or even a rolling pin from the kitchen.

BAFENG ("BA-FUNG"), EIGHT WINDS

Why to do it: The feet are an especially sensitive, often neglected, area of the body. Applying pressure to the Bafeng point, or as it is translated in the West, the Eight Winds, can reduce feelings of depression or sadness not uncommon in the postnatal period.

How to do it: From a seated position, take one foot in your hands. With the top of your foot facing up toward you, notice the webs of skin between your toes. Using your index finger and thumb, begin by gently pinching the area of skin between your big toe and your second toe. Spend a few seconds gently rubbing the area and then proceed to do the same with each of the webbed spaces between the remaining toes. Be sure to spend some time on both feet. Happy feet will take a mama a long way.

SMALL INTESTINE 1

Why to do it: Practitioners of acupuncture and acupressure believe this point can promote lactation.

How to do it: On each pinky finger, about one quarter of an inch below the cuticle (toward the knuckle) and slightly toward the outside of the arm (away from the thumb), lies the point known as the Small Intestine 1. Using a fingernail or even the tip of a ballpoint pen, apply pressure to the point. This is a naturally sensitive area. A soreness will be felt at the sight even when slight pressure is applied there. Spend about thirty seconds on each pinky and aim for twice daily.

SPLEEN 6

Why to do it: Treating the Spleen 6 point can be an effective way to relieve postpartum uterine cramping. This point can help the uterus to contract more efficiently after birth, and in so doing shrink the organ to its normal size. Some find that treating this point can help the body to rebuild blood supply and restore energy levels.

How to do it: From the tip of the inner ankle bone, the Spleen 6 point may be found four fingers up (closer to the head) on the inside of the leg. A slight depression may be felt at the site. Gentle pressure applied with the thumb may result in some initial soreness, but this should dissipate rather quickly. Hold your thumb on the point for thirty seconds to a minute. Be sure to treat the point on both legs, one at a time. Treating both sides will increase effectiveness. Steer clear of treating the Spleen 6 point during pregnancy as doing so may stimulate contractions. In fact, the point is often treated to help initiate labor! Also skip the point if there is excessive postpartum bleeding or hemorrhage.

STOMACH 36, LEG 3 MILES

Why to do it: Moms who are feeling weak or sore following labor and delivery will welcome some attention to the Stomach 36 point. Similar to Spleen 6, some believe that treating this point, also referred to as Leg 3 Miles, can boost energy.

How to do it: From a seated position, locate the patella or kneecap. Place one hand just below the bone and slightly to the outside away from the body. Your hand should be just at the top edge of the tibia, the larger of the two lower leg bones. Using your thumb, rub the area in a clockwise direction for thirty seconds to a minute on each side. A feeling of mild soreness or warmth may emerge in the area. You may treat both sides simultaneously or one and then the other, as it feels comfortable for you.

STOMACH QI-POINTS, STOMACH QI-LINE

Why to do it: Beginning just below the knee and ending just above the ankle, most people will observe a series of hard, lumpy spots. In acupuncture and acupressure, these points are understood to impact digestion, as they affect stomach Qi. Treating these points may help with stomach ailments and with keeping things moving. Some people have one or two of these spots while others have several, and the amount and number of spots tend to vary between the right and left legs.

How to do it: Using your thumb or fingertip, place a finger just below the knee and begin to slowly slide down until a hard spot is felt. Hold and press, applying pressure downward in the direction of the heel, for about thirty seconds. The spot may feel a bit sore at first and then should begin to soften. Continue sliding down until the next spot is detected and then repeat until all spots have been massaged. Be sure to try and do both legs. You may treat both at once or one after the other.

STOMACH 13

Why to do it: Growing and carrying a baby is a tall order, and it can leave a mother's body pretty worn down—literally. The Stomach 13 point can help by lifting the body back up! Treating this area can aid in straightening up the lower abdominal region, which is drawn out and down with the weight of a pregnancy. It can also be used to combat feelings of fatigue and heaviness in the legs. Attending to the Stomach 13 point may be helpful if there is any sort of sinking feeling in the perineum, the area between the vagina and the anus. Women who have an episiotomy, a surgical incision to widen the opening for birth, or who experienced any tearing during labor may find particular relief.

Practitioners will also treat the Stomach 13 point in cases of uterine prolapse. This can occur when the muscles that support the uterus become weakened (following labor, for example) and slip down from their usual position. Backaches, as well as discomfort in the groin area, may also be alleviated by treating this point.

How to do it: Just below the collarbone, halfway between the midline of the body and the tip of the shoulder, there is a small depression or "knot." This area has a "gummy" feel to it and is often rather tender. Using any fingertip, press into the area moving out and up toward the shoulder. Think of the motion of straightening a shirt on a hanger. Do not actually slide your fingertip up, but rather apply pressure in the direction of the shoulder tip. Be sure to treat both sides, aiming for thirty seconds to a minute on each side. Tension should begin to soften and tenderness will dissipate.

HEART 3

Why to do it: The privilege of motherhood is usually accompanied by the responsibility of primary caregiver. Constant care-giving necessitates that one's mind, body, and spirit be replenished. This is where sending a little love to the Heart 3 point can be especially helpful. The point is known to generally calm the spirit and relieve tension in the neck and the low back. Breastfeeding moms may find treating this area to be especially helpful in relieving the tension that results from hunching over to nurse.

How to do it: Extend your hand and arm out, palm upward, with a slight bend in the elbow. Place the thumb of your opposite hand on the elbow crease and slide it gently downward toward the bony portion of the elbow. Between the end of the crease and this bony area is a meaty, fleshy bit of skin where the Heart 3 point resides. Apply pressure to this area for thirty seconds to a minute. Any tension should begin to soften as pressure is applied. Repeat on the other side.

A NOTE ON AURICULAR ACUPRESSURE

Beyond listening to baby's coos and cries, a mother's ears are a thing of beauty and they should be treated accordingly. Auricular, or ear, acupressure can be restorative in the postpartum period. The meridian points on the ear are small and be can be challenging to identify on one's own. Misidentifying a point can be ineffective and frustrating—no good. In lieu of performing ear treatments on yourself, consider stimulating the area using essential oil. Lavender oil, known as shen men or "spirit gate," can be used topically on the skin and may have a calming and relaxing effect. On the upper part of the ear is a fleshy triangular area known as the triangular fossa. This is a slightly indented dip just beneath the harder cartilage ridge at the top. Rub a drop of oil between the fingertips and then apply gently to the area.

While acupressure is easily performed on oneself, it can also be a wonderful activity to engage in with a co-parent. A partner

While acupressure is easily performed on oneself, it can also be a wonderful activity to engage in with a co-parent. can administer acupressure using the same techniques you might use on yourself. Working as a pair, the practice can be enhanced by synchronizing your breathing. Registered nurse and certified childbirth educator Sherry L. M. Jiménéz writes that focusing on a rhythmic image, such as a pendulum swinging back and forth, can help to regulate the breath and aid couples in connecting with each other. Doing so can deepen the practice and enhance the overall experience (Jimenez 1995, 7–10).

Acupressure can be a wonderful mechanism for healing and promoting overall wellness during the postpartum phase and beyond, though there are a number of contraindications. In addition to those noted on each particular point outlined earlier, the following should also be considered: Those with blood clots should not employ these techniques. Mothers who have diabetes or other conditions that affect sensation in the feet or other part of the body should not practice acupressure. If there is an infection or swelling, cuts or scrapes, or damage to the skin on a point, do not apply acupressure to the area. Finally, acupressure should not be used over a broken bone or damaged nerve or organ. If you're uncertain, it may be useful to have at least one initial consultation with an experienced practitioner before using self- or partner-administered treatment. See the Resources section in the back of the book to find a local professional.

Acupressure can be an effective, easy-to-practice support at this time in life and moving forward. Ashley Flores advises her clients to "listen to their fingers," when practicing on themselves. New mothers must be allowed the time to turn their attention to their own bodies. Whether pregnancy was easy or complex, whether labor was natural or required interventions, what is certain is that the body has been through an extraordinary series of events. Mothers who became so through adoption may have experienced the psychological and physical stressors of fertility treatments that failed, not to mention the challenges of the adoption process itself. Whatever your path to motherhood, your body is likely to bear the scars of that journey. Listen to your fingers. Let them guide you toward a place of healing.

Just as acupressure can work to stimulate the flow of Qi in the body, creating art can work to stimulate the flow of emotion and expression—and the health implications for mothers and babies are both tangible and extraordinary. Think this is traditional arts and crafts? Think again.

EXPRESSIVE-ARTS THERAPY

MORE THAN ARTS & CRAFTS

Art washes away from the soul the dust of everyday life.

—Pablo Picasso, Spanish painter

I f they are lucky, children in primary school take art class as part of a weekly schedule. There is (or, at least, there should be) ample opportunity to play, to get messy, and to express oneself in an open and carefree way. As children grow, unless they are drawn (no pun intended) to art and supported in the endeavor, designated time to create is often replaced by pursuits that society deems more productive, acceptable, or financially reliable. With maturity also comes the realization that art is evaluated by others.

Is it well done? Is it an investment piece? Unfortunately, the value of creating for the sake of creating is often lost.

Deciding to make art as an adult, and specifically at this moment in life, can be powerful and transformative. Multiple studies point to the therapeutic benefits of expressive-arts therapy for both mothers and their infants. Over the last decade, a body of research demonstrates the healing effects of art-making in bolstering maternal self-esteem and facilitating mother-infant bonding.

In the same way it is beneficial to exercise the body at this time (more on this in the chapter "Flexercise: How a Little Workout Can Go a Long Way") exercising one's creativity also promotes health and healing, according to registered social worker and expressive-arts therapist Kaeli Macdonald (pers. comm.). When feeling stuck in the day-to-day tasks of postpartum life, art therapy can be a way to stimulate change and realize that change is indeed possible. In beginning with a blank canvas or a blank page, you are free to build something original, something exclusively of your own design. Letting creativity take the lead can help us access and release deep emotion. Doing so can be remarkably therapeutic.

In the work of mothering, how often do you feel unable to control a given situation? If you're like most of us, the answer is probably somewhere in the countless-times-a-day range. Many women experience this loss of control as early as the birth process, with the sensation of giving in to the force of one's body. For other mothers, control is usurped, as may be the case if a medical intervention is required or suggested.

Mothers who have a relatively smooth labor and delivery might first encounter this particular lack of command in the first weeks postpartum, when baby's eating and sleeping habits are erratic. Still others will feel the pinch during toddlerhood, when temperaments can be fickle and tantrums can swell. Being an art-maker can bring relief in all of these instances because it provides something very special: the chance to play the role of director. This position—the director, the maker—brings with it the freedom to design every aspect of a project. You can choose what medium to use, what colors, and when it is complete. You can pause to assess. You can design and mold and shape as you go. The maker can "titrate the pace" of her own craft, as Kaeli Macdonald puts it. For moms who are feeling a shortage of order or reliability in their daily lives, art therapy affords you a chance to reclaim it—if only for a short time.

Besides the chance to sit in the director's chair, art can also serve as a way to recognize and communicate deep emotion for which language may feel inadequate. Even the most eloquent people have moments when speech is ineffective or incomplete. Remember the expression "a picture is worth a thousand words"? Especially at times of heightened emotion—anger and frustration, elation and bliss—art captures feelings in a way that words cannot. Art therapy is a pathway to healing when words fail. Since babies have not yet developed their language skills, making art together can connect you and your baby without the need for verbal communication.

A RETREAT FROM THE REAL WORLD:
ALLISON'S STORY

I was never artistic. I took a painting class in college to fulfill an arts requirement, but that's about it. The class was kind of fun. I didn't make a masterpiece, but I did find the act of painting pretty relaxing. I could kind of zone out during the brush strokes and clear my head a bit; it was a nice escape from my everyday stress. So, when I noticed the local YMCA was offering an art class for mothers and their babies, I thought it might be worth checking out. Brian was one year old at the time and the year had been rough for me. I just hadn't been myself since he was born. The class was small and pretty laid back—just two other moms and their kids, the art teacher, and an early childhood specialist attended. The art teacher was wonderful. She was very encouraging and supportive and made the space feel really comfortable. Together with the specialist, we were taught how to work with our babies in painting together. It almost felt like a retreat from the real world. For that hour once a week, I was able to be with my baby doing something different than the usual nursing, changing, and sleeping routine.

The American Art Therapy Association defines art therapy as "an integrative mental health and human services profession that enriches the lives of individuals, families, and communities through active art-making, creative process, applied psychological theory, and human experience within a psychotherapeutic relationship" (2017, par. 2). Art therapy can help people become better in touch with their feelings, resolve emotional conflicts, deepen self-awareness, manage behavior, lower anxiety, and boost self-esteem. Given the challenges inherent in early motherhood, the feasibility and accessibility of art therapy make it an excellent tool to add to the box. This is not about making great art. No special skills or previous experience are required to engage in or benefit from these activities. All that is needed is an openness to explore the possibility.

Art therapy can help people become better in touch with their feelings, resolve emotional conflicts, deepen self-awareness, manage behavior, lower anxiety, and boost self-esteem.

A small UK-based study published in the *International Journal of Art Therapy* looked at the healing impact of a twenty-week painting group for new mothers and their little ones. The researchers specifically studied the effect of participation on maternal self-esteem, depression, and mother-infant bonding. Researchers noted that participants' self-esteem had risen an average of 70 percent and depressive feelings were reduced! Who wouldn't want to feel 70 percent better about herself, mother or no? A measure of the quality of the mother-infant relationship had improved by 63 percent over the baseline at the start of the study. Observers of the group noticed the mother-child relationship growing closer as they painted together. Some of the more intimate moments were documented in photographs, which were then given to the mothers as mementos of the artistic journey they shared together (Hosea 2006, 69–78).

Renowned pediatrician and psychoanalyst Donald Winnicott writes of the importance of establishing a *potential space* between a mother and her baby. This concept refers to an imagined area in which the two share in creative and relaxed play (1971). Imagine an orchestra in the moment before the conductor moves his baton to signal the start of an overture. Or sitting in a theatre just after the light dims and before the show begins or the curtain goes up. There is a very particular energy that can be felt: a special quality in the ether that suggests something is about to be created—birthed. This same environment can be created between you and your baby. This potential space is a prime opportunity to enhance communication and healthy relationship building. Painting together is a way of making room for this very space. By affording a safe, welcome escape from the challenges of early child-rearing, you can relate in a new way to both your baby and yourself. Between birth and age three, the kind of attachment a child makes with her mother or primary caregiver is profound. The quality of that first relationship has lasting implications for all the relationships that follow, establishing a model upon which all others will be based. This unique time is the perfect time to create both art and strong family bonds.

PAINTING AS A PATH TO CONNECTION: NANCEY'S STORY

I always assumed that I would fall in love with my baby as soon as I laid eyes on her. It didn't happen that way. When Ava was born, I remember the nurse putting her in my arms and thinking, "Who is this little person? She isn't really mine, is she!?" It was weird. I just didn't feel the overwhelming love I hear other moms talk about. For a while, I really thought something was wrong with me. Ava was an adorable baby—everyone said so. She was smiley and sweet, but it was like I couldn't connect with her. I became more and more upset—depressed really—believing that I was never going to be the mother she deserved.

In grad school, I used to paint on the weekends. I would take a small easel, paints, and a canvas out to the park and paint for hours. When Ava was about ten months old, I was feeding her some vanilla pudding. She loved it so much she just put four fingers in the bowl and right into her mouth. Then she wiped them on the tray of her high chair, leaving a small trace of the pudding behind. Suddenly, I was reminded about painting. I made some edible finger paint using yogurt and we started painting together. I'm not sure who loved it more—me or Ava. For the first time, I felt like this is my daughter, no doubt about it.

Art therapist Hilary Hosea comments on the powerful symbolism of art created for the purpose of healing. She remarks that "paintings themselves often become objects . . . invested with the power to carry the relationship between mother and infant forward in a more optimistic and hopeful way" (Arroyo and Fowler 2013, 102). In the UK art therapy group mentioned earlier, the meaningfulness of the paintings created was underscored by those mothers who chose to showcase the work in their homes. Though the objective of the group was not to make decorative art, the canvases captured such powerful symbolism—the evolution of the mother-infant relationship—that mothers wanted this to be witnessed.

Beyond bonding with their babies, mothers in the group also found themselves bonding with one another. As the weeks progressed, participants became more willing to open up about their own experiences. Social isolation, stress, illness, and divorce were some of the topics individuals explored in the art room. Researchers speculated that perhaps mothers were willing to expose such common vulnerabilities because the group was not designed to be talk therapy (Arroyo and Fowler 2013, 102). Free of the stigma that sometimes accompanies more traditional support groups, the art room provided an invitation not just to express creativity, but to express feelings openly, as well. Imagine the value of having a place to go, to play, to share your experiences of motherhood fully, without fear of judgment or ridicule. Can you imagine the impact on your life?

As with most of the tools in this book, art therapy is effective for mothers to engage in with or without their babies. A second UK-based study followed a different group, Time For Me, established for mothers of children aged two and younger. Group participants reported experiencing mild to moderate depression and anxiety in relation to becoming moms. The objective of Time for Me was to create a comfortable space, bolster self-esteem through the arts, and reduce feelings of social isolation that often accompany this time in life. The group met weekly for eight, ninety-minute sessions and included activities like card-making, collage, and ceramics. At the conclusion, interviews with the participating mothers indicated they felt greater

Imagine the value of having a place to go, to play, to share your experiences of motherhood fully, without fear of judgment or ridicule.

confidence and self-esteem (Perry, Thurston, and Osborn, 2008, 1438–45). This may have come in part from the sense of accomplishment in creating and completing a tangible product—of being in that director's chair.

Support groups, be they art-based or not, are a popular therapeutic model because they can offer a sense of camaraderie, social support, and validation. Art therapy groups have the added benefit of allowing a participant to work independently while being surrounded by others in similar circumstances. In creating one's own art within the context of a group setting, a mom can enjoy a special opportunity for self-reflection amongst like-minded others. Further, art therapy groups can be an inspiring way to meet and connect with people. Whereas language is typically our primary form of connection, making art together communicates parts of ourselves we don't often readily share.

If the idea of joining a group appeals to you, find out if the local YMCA, community center, or college has an art therapist on staff and ask to speak with her. Or, check out the Resources section in the back of the book to contact the American Art Therapy Association to locate a professional in your area. Some moms may be lucky enough to find mother-infant art groups where they live. If a group is not available or you'd like to try a one-on-one experience, consider working with a licensed creative or expressive-arts therapist. This is someone who has education and experience in using the arts (fine arts, music, movement, writing, or drama) for a therapeutic purpose.

Whether or not an art therapy group or art therapist sounds like a good fit, there are simple exercises that you can try on your own. Before doing so, consider which exercise(s) to choose and identify specific goals. What do you hope to gain from using this tool? Is the purpose to find a different way to connect with your baby? Or to add some variety into the daily routine? Perhaps you are looking to shift the focus onto yourself (Hooray!). Maybe you are feeling anxious or sad but cannot seem to verbalize why? Maybe you are having trouble knowing exactly what you're feeling? (Sounds like motherhood, in a nutshell.) Considering these questions can help in selecting the activities detailed below. These techniques come by way of Kaeli Macdonald, who provides support to pre- and postnatal clients in Canada.

> Whereas language is typically our primary form of connection, making art together communicates parts of ourselves we don't often readily share.

VISUAL JOURNAL/VISION BOARD

Why to do it: In the same way that one might keep a written journal or diary to express her innermost thoughts, a vision journal or vision board can achieve the same objective through pictures or images instead of words. If your goal is to identify and explore your feelings, this is a wonderful tool. A vision board can also be used to create an image that represents how you *wish* things might be. For example, if you are longing for the day (or night) when your little one is sleeping more regularly, you may be moved by images of people at rest or in a state of relaxation. Creating a tangible document of your hopes for the future can be deeply empowering and afford some sense of relief in the midst of a challenging present.

How to do it: This activity is best done in a twenty- to thirty-minute window of time alone. If your baby is on a somewhat reliable nap schedule, seize the chance to try out the exercise. Begin by clearing a space to work. You will need a large sheet of paper or artist's sketch book, as well as newspapers, magazines, scissors, and glue. Have markers or colored pencils on hand as well. Take a couple of moments to focus on your breath. With your eyes closed, expand the breathing so that air is taken deep into the diaphragm. This will help to increase relaxation before beginning your creative process. Flip through the magazines and newspapers and observe the pictures. Follow what art therapists call the *sense base*, not the *practical base*. Try and turn down the volume of the thinking brain and, instead, be led by feelings rather than thoughts. Tear or cut out any images that resonate in some way. Try not to think about what images you are choosing or why. Do not judge or censor. Affix the pictures to the paper in whatever way feels right (knowing of course that there is no real right or wrong).

When you're finished (or when your baby wakes up), place your creation somewhere safe and let it rest for a while. Notice if your feelings at the start of the exercise are any different from those at its completion. Make a note of it, either on the back page of the artwork itself or in a separate notebook. See the Templates section in the back of this book for an example. The option always exists to revisit the work again. When observed some time later, this kind of art should be viewed more like a diary entry, not like a painting in a museum. What does the image convey? How does it feel? Does it offer any insight into the experience you were having when you made it? "Vision boards may demonstrate who [you are] as a mom now, or the mother [you] would like to be," points out Kaeli Macdonald (pers. comm.).

WATCH, WAIT & WONDER

Why to do it: Ever unsure of how to engage with your little one? Of course you are! At times we all are. Never in the history, or rather herstory, of mom-kind has a mother known just what to say or do around her baby at every moment. So often, new moms feel at a loss for what to *do* with their little ones beyond the routine tasks of feeding and diaper-changing. If your goal is to spice things up in your daily mothercare routine, then Watch, Wait & Wonder is the way to go. This exercise is used both in art therapy groups and also in individual therapist/client sessions as a technique that can help a mother connect more deeply with her baby in a fun and pressure-free way. This activity has the added advantage of helping us to see our children as truly separate individuals, and also to help create a deeper understanding of our own emotional responses to our children's behaviors.

How to do it: Watch, Wait & Wonder works best with a child who is six months or older. In this exercise, your child takes the lead. Begin by setting up a safe space to explore. If there is a rug on the floor roll it up or cover it with a plastic tarp or something to protect the surface. Choose a variety of art materials, making sure, of course, that they are non-toxic and safe for use with young children. Certain food-based products can substitute for paint. For example, Jell-O powder in yogurt makes a paint-like substance in different colors. Raw vegetables like potatoes or apples can be cut into shapes and used as stamps. Have a variety of paint brushes on hand. Then, simply sit on the floor with your baby. In this exercise, you are the attentive observer and your child is the art-maker. Do not feel compelled to *do* anything. (What a relief!) Instead, use the time to observe how your baby behaves in the artistic space. Try not to assume what he wants. For instance, your little one may hand you a brush. Rather than starting to paint with it (a natural impulse), what if you simply accept this gift and then watch to see what he does next? Enjoy being free of the pressure to do. Simply observe. Are there colors to which he seems attracted? Does he appear engaged? Uninterested?

In observing your child, be mindful of your own internal responses. What feelings are being generated? Are you calmer and more relaxed? Are you anxious about baby making a mess? Or having to clean it up? No judgment here! For the purposes of this activity, your responses to your baby's actions are just as important as the actions themselves. *Every* feeling is valid. Remember, this is all about getting to know yourself better as a mother, as well as getting to know your baby in a new way. Be aware and be together. Enjoy the discovery!

ONE-LINE JOURNAL

Why to do it: There are days when you barely have time to pee let alone set up an art studio. There are days when your baby won't sleep or is colicky or is just fussy no matter what you do. These are the days when the one-line journal can be your best friend. The goal here is to provide a quick outlet for releasing strong emotion when time and energy are in short supply. Getting emotion out of the body and onto paper, even with only a brief moment to pause and express it, can provide a surprising sense of relief.

How to do it: Reserve a legal pad exclusively for this purpose, or simply take a piece of notebook paper or whatever is on hand and convenient. Grab a marker or a crayon and fill up a line or two. Scribble, draw an image, letters, words, a pattern—anything that comes out. This should be a quick burst of creativity, rather than one that is carefully executed. Once you've got the words out, you can decide what to do with the page. Some moms like to keep it, so they can reflect back and explore the content more deeply at another time. Others revel in the opportunity to crumple it up and toss it away: one step further in releasing the feelings.

Getting emotion out of the body and onto paper, even with only a brief moment to pause and express it, can provide a surprising sense of relief.

MOLD THE DOUGH

Why to do it: Unlike paint (unless it is finger paint), crayons, or markers, working in clay or Play-Doh necessitates that one's hands be immersed in the material. As a result, clay can provide a unique, multi-sensory experience. For some, the medium enables a more complete vehicle for emotional expression. Mold the Dough is the go-to exercise for moms who like to get their hands dirty, so to speak. At one time, most of us loved that feeling. This may explain why many a second-grader comes home from school at some point during the year with a clay object vaguely resembling a coffee mug. (The most beautiful coffee mug ever, right?)

How to do it: A bit of time, space, and clay or Play-Doh are all that is needed. Let your hands mold the material. Take the time to step back and look at your work as you go, being sure to take advantage of the three-dimensional aspect of the clay. Unlike other mediums, clay can be viewed from all angles, so be sure to rotate your piece looking at various angles from the top, bottom, and sides. Remember to lower the volume on your thinking brain and let your emotions guide you. Try putting on some classical or other lyric-free music in the background while you create. This can help quiet the thoughts and amplify what is happening emotionally.

COLORING BOOK

Why to do it: Though people often think about coloring books for children, they can be a useful tool for adults as well. In fact, select adult coloring books are now among Amazon's best-sellers, and Crayola, the king of crayon-makers, has recently launched a line of markers, pencils, and coloring books aimed at the adult market. If the idea of art therapy seems abstract or difficult, using a coloring book can be a good place to begin. Putting color to paper can accomplish three goals: to help reluctant artists acclimate to the idea of art therapy, to aid in stress relief, and to create expression in its own right.

How to do it: Children are usually instructed to color within the lines. What would happen if you were given permission to color outside of them? In your coloring book, indulge in breaking free of the mold. See what happens creatively when you are not bound by the rigid confines of those thick black boundaries. The actual coloring book is not especially important, though the subject matter should be of interest. As an option, deepen the experience by adding to the image being colored. Consider using the coloring book page as a foundation and build a collage on top of it (more on this next). Play with layering, a metaphor for the layered emotions of your personal motherhood experience.

COLLAGE

Why to do it: Creating a collage serves as a useful alternative or complement to painting. Collage-making is even easier in the sense that it requires fewer materials (no paint or paintbrushes) and less clean up. Collages offer tremendous creative freedom in that space can be expanded by using extra paper or by building up the layers. A collage is similar to a vision board, as they are both a collection of images. However, the goal for a collage is somewhat different. In making a collage, you have the opportunity to focus on a particular theme in your maternal experience. You might choose to design a piece that reflects how you are feeling about the changes in your body, for example, or the shift in your relationship with your partner or your own mother. A collage allows you to be more focused on your emotional expression of a specific aspect of your life at this moment in time.

How to do it: Use as many or as few materials as you wish. The only essentials required are paper, glue, and magazines. You can add other materials like fabric, corrugated paper, string, or buttons—anything goes! Flip through the pages of the magazine and cut or tear out those images, shapes, and colors that resonate with your chosen theme. Glue them and your other materials on the paper as you select them, or gather them all first and then glue them on at the end. As an alternative (or in addition), feel free to draw and color your own images, if you are so inspired, and add these to the collage. Notice any feelings coming up while moving through the process. Are certain images eliciting any particular emotions? Remember, there is always the freedom to stop, take a break, and come back to your artwork at a later time.

There are only a few instances when art therapy is contraindicated. If you are experiencing severe depression or anxiety or hallucinations or delusions, art therapy is not a sufficient source of support on its own. In these cases, more immediate treatment is required, usually in the form of talk therapy and perhaps medication too. (See the chapter "Talk Is *Not* Cheap: The Value of Talk Therapy" for more.) If you are having these symptoms, please call your healthcare provider right away. Reliable treatment is available and you are entitled to and deserving of it.

As with many therapies—talk, art, or otherwise—sometimes the process leaves people feeling worse before they feel better. Unexpected, sometimes unpleasant, emotions may come to the surface during the creative process. If it feels like too much, leave the art alone. Step away for a day or two and come back around with a set of fresh eyes. Or reach out to a therapist who can help.

You can also consider working with a different kind of medium. While the focus here is on the visual arts, expressive-arts therapists often work in multiple modalities including music, dance, and drama. Some moms will have a stronger connection to these other art forms. Check out the Resources section in the back of this book for more information.

If art therapy leaves you hungry for more, or maybe just hungry, read on! Learn about how food, the oldest form of medicine, can feed a whole lot more than just the body.

FEED ME!

HEALING MEALS FOR MAMAS

Let food be thy medicine and medicine be thy food.

—Hippocrates, Greek physician

This chapter is not about losing the baby weight. For most new moms, pound-shedding is already on their to-do list somewhere between laundry loads and washing breast pump parts. Because so many of us cannot escape the overwhelming pressure to don the skinny jeans ASAP (more than a few pregnant women have packed a pair in the hospital bag—wishful thinking), included later in the chapter are some tried and true tips for weight loss. Really though, the main purpose here is to reconsider one's relationship with food at this unique moment in life, assess whether or not it is working, and learn how to make this relationship better. This chapter is about not only what a mom eats, but also *how* she eats.

LEARNING HOW TO EAT

Dieting is not the answer to lasting weight loss and it certainly does not do much for mood. (I've never wanted a piece of chocolate cake more than when I felt I couldn't have one!) Recently, *The New York Times* chronicled a long list of winning contestants on the reality TV show *The Biggest Loser*, all of whom had regained some of, all of, or more than the weight they lost once upon a time in TV land. These folks had a cadre of professional health and fitness folks at their disposal, not to mention millions of viewers witnessing their progress from the comfort of their living rooms. Still, this was not enough to make the weight loss last well beyond the season finale. Lest there be any doubt that losing and keeping weight off is a formidable task, the proof is in the proverbial pudding.

The process of becoming a mother and incorporating this new identity is a perfect time to contemplate your eating habits and food choices. Just as you are learning to feed your baby, whether by breast, bottle, or both, you can also take this opportunity to learn or perhaps *re*learn how to feed yourself. Eating, though it is something most of us do multiple times a day, is an act few of us are actually taught to do in an optimal way. While people need to eat to live, the way they think about eating, or, more often, do not think about it, can have profound effects on physical and emotional health. The food that is available to us and our observations of others' eating habits, especially when we're young, greatly influence our patterns of behavior. How we interact

Eating, though it is something most of us do multiple times a day, is an act few of us are actually taught to do in an optimal way.

with the contents of the refrigerator, the pantry, and the take-out menu is often based on what has been modeled for us—the good, the bad, and the ugly.

During the postpartum stage, the dietary choices mothers make are arguably more important than those they have made in the past. At this moment, a new mom has a unique opportunity to learn about and adopt a healthy relationship with food and then model it for her child. This is a precious, potentially life-long gift for both a mom and her baby.

Suppose that instead of thinking about eating to lose weight, as is commonly done in the months following birth, you were to think about the act of eating itself. To be more specific, the *way* you eat. Eating habits are very particular. One person may tend to eat very slowly, while another is often the first to finish what is on her plate (that would be me). Then there are multitasking-eaters: those who check email, read, or send a text while chewing. Some people are grazers, snacking throughout the day, while others tend to eat a more traditional breakfast, lunch, and dinner.

Begin to pay attention to your eating patterns. Notice if your eating tends to be associated with particular emotions—happiness, sadness, fatigue, or boredom. Try to observe patterns without judgment. There is no need to form an opinion about your personal behaviors, especially if it is a negative one. Instead, simply think about seeking the answers as something of an exploratory mission: a chance to learn more deeply about yourself. If you need a strong motivation to better understand your interaction with food, consider this: the way you eat can be a healing force.

The effectiveness of mindfulness-based interventions in eating is a research specialty of Dr. Jane Hart, Clinical Instructor and former Chair of the Integrative Medicine Committee at Case Western Reserve University School of Medicine in Cleveland, Ohio. She has seen improvements in weight loss, decreases in

If you need a strong motivation to better understand your interaction with food, consider this: the way you eat can be a healing force.

eating disorders, and reductions in food cravings, through the use of a mindfulness-based approach. Dr. Hart comments that " . . . how, when, and why a person eats may be just as important as what that person eats to optimize his or her health" (2014, 317). Researchers at the University of Oxford Mindfulness Center recently teamed up with the maternity division of Oxford University hospitals to implement the Mindfulness-Based Childbirth and Parenting Program (MBCP) with pre- and postnatal patients. The team reported that "teaching mindfulness in the perinatal period seems to have the effect of broadening women's personal repertoire of coping strategies, and this has potential to improve the developmental trajectory of parents and infants" (Warriner, Dymond, and Williams 2013, 521).

So, what is mindfulness exactly? More specifically, what is a mindfulness-based approach to eating? Though not a religious practice, the idea of mindfulness draws on traditional Buddhist meditation practices dating back more than two thousand years. Mindfulness places focus on awareness and keeping attention in the present moment. (We will explore this idea more fully in the chapter "Meditation: Om Away the Baby Blues and Some Other Things Too.") When it comes to eating, a mindfulness-based approach offers that the act should incorporate the senses and be performed with purpose. In the hectic day-to-day life of a new mother, eating is seldom an activity unto itself. More often, eating is conducted in conjunction with other activities—checking a Twitter feed or Instagram account, or even while traveling from a play group to a play date. Mindful eating is meant to be its *own* pursuit, performed thoughtfully and singularly.

How might mindful eating look in practice? Imagine this: A simple bowl of penne pasta with marinara sauce sits on a table. Whereas one's impulse (like mine) might be to dive headfirst into the mound of tubular goodness, instead one chooses to pause for a moment. External distractions are limited. A cell phone is silenced, the laptop is closed, and baby is placed in the bouncer. Then, the chunks of juicy tomato shimmering in the sauce are observed. One indulges in a deep breath in through the nose, inhaling the garlic and oregano-infused steam. Salivating yet? The experience could even be verbalized and shared with your baby. "This pasta smells soooo yummy! The steam feels like a little kiss on my nose." Gracefully, the hollow noodle is slipped onto the spear of the fork as the sauce clings to its edges. Slowly, the fork meets the mouth as the warm and tender pasta slides onto the tongue and the Parmesan flakes melt. This, in a nutshell, is mindful eating. In limiting distractions, you are free to draw attention more fully to the food you are about to enjoy. Utilizing all the senses expands the experience of eating, making it more of a pleasurable activity, not simply a necessity.

Eating in a mindful way offers the added advantage of slowing down the meal. This can have real implications for weight loss and weight management. When we eat quickly, we deprive our digestive and nervous systems of the chance to communicate with one another. It takes about twenty minutes for the brain to regi ster that the stomach is feeling full. Eating quickly increases the likelihood of overeating. No one should be expected to be able to sit down on a daily basis for a leisurely two-hour lunch (at least, no one who has any idea what early childcare entails), but the principle of pace-setting in a realistic way can be modified to work

Utilizing all the senses expands the experience of eating, making it more of a pleasurable activity, not simply a necessity.

for moms. Even by placing baby in his bassinet or swing for ten minutes—five even—and employing all the maternal senses to focus solely on the meal at hand, your dining experience can be transformed. The result may be a more relaxing experience and perhaps one that requires less food to feel sated.

MAKING MORE OF MEALTIME: ABIGAIL'S STORY

Food and I have never had the easiest of relationships. I was chunky growing up and always a little self-conscious about my weight. In my mid-twenties, I lost about ten pounds and was the most content with my weight that I had ever been. This is why, when I became pregnant at thirty, I was both elated and anxious about what it would mean to gain that weight back—and then some. More so, I was concerned about how I would look and feel about my weight after my daughter was born. Somewhere late in my pregnancy, I realized that I wanted to try and make sure my daughter had a healthier attitude around eating than I had. I met with a nutritionist who helped me design a meal plan for the remainder of my pregnancy, while breastfeeding, and beyond. More than the food itself, though, she spoke with me about changing my eating habits. As often as possible, she encouraged me to make meal times something of a sacred activity—free from interruptions and distractions. To be honest, it took some getting used to, and I didn't always want to do it. I was used to eating in front of the TV or my laptop. Eventually though, I got more used to focusing only on the food in front of me. Of course, I'm not able to treat every meal as its own event, especially now that my daughter is two, but I am able to do so for some of my meals. Not only is this way of eating more peaceful, but it helps me control my weight too. I always seem to feel more satisfied when I eat consciously.

Registered dietitian, exercise physiologist, and New York City–based personal trainer Mary Jane Detroyer suggests that mindfulness can be helpful in food selection as well. Picking which foods to eat in a mindful way encourages taking the time to recognize and honor one's feelings. "Choosing to eat emotionally is very different than eating without awareness," says Detroyer (pers. comm.). She encourages her clients to try and be more adept at recognizing their internal cues about eating. Before opening the refrigerator for example, you might ask, "Am I feeling hungry now, or am I feeling something else?" Though everyone has experienced the sensation of hunger, sometimes it can be difficult to distinguish this from other feelings, like anxiety or stress. Cultivating an awareness of why and when you are choosing to eat a particular food can be empowering, enabling you to seize greater control of your choices.

Detroyer suggests using a food journal to help recognize eating habits. This does not have to be a complex record of everything you consume (there's no mama-time for that anyway). See the Templates section in the back of this book for a simple option that may be copied and kept on or near the refrigerator. You can also use a white board or kitchen chalkboard—whatever feels most comfortable for you. Before opening the fridge, take a moment for an emotional inventory. Notice any feelings coming up and write them down. Ask yourself: Is there something going on here besides hunger? This simple question can create a sense of awareness and may stop an act of mindless eating before it starts. It is possible that writing down the feelings may actually replace the urge to swallow them with food. Now that's power! Of course, if the feeling you've written down truly *is* hunger, by all means, enjoy the gift of food.

Start becoming more aware of personal eating patterns. Simply noticing them can begin the process of small changes that, in time, can have a big impact on the food relationship. Be realistic and patient. On some days there will not be time to make lunch, let alone eat it mindfully. That's okay. Baby steps.

LEARNING WHAT TO EAT

Now that we have a better idea about *how* to eat, let's consider *what* we can bring to the table to optimize our overall health. Food is another tool that can positively impact postpartum healing.

Different foods can be used to affect many of the complex physical and psychological shifts that come after giving birth. From exhaustion to mood swings, food can serve as a powerful antidote to some of the most frequent hardships new mothers encounter. A crash course in what to eat can go a long way toward feeling better, faster.

FATIGUE

One of the most grueling aspects of new motherhood is managing the period of time before your little one catches on to the fact that days are for waking and nights are for sleeping. For many moms, getting through the day with so little sleep at night is the most arduous part of mothering in the early days. Thankfully, the foods you opt for can make a difference in helping cope with a chronic case of the *Zzzzs*. One of the best

From exhaustion to mood swings, food can serve as a powerful antidote to some of the most frequent hardships new mothers encounter.

ways to stave off physical and emotional fatigue nutritionally is to keep blood sugar levels even throughout the day, according to Nutritional Therapist Patricia Gilroy. She offers that complex carbohydrates such as whole wheat bread, whole wheat pasta, and brown rice are preferable to their white counterparts, which can lead to a rapid spike and drop in levels. A tall glass of water along with those carbs is also a good idea. Water can keep bodily systems running smoothly and reduce the risk of constipation—a common culprit of fatigue (Gilroy 2016).

Anemia can also result in tiredness. Not unusual in pregnancy, this condition is the result of a lack of healthy red blood cells needed to carry oxygen throughout the body. In cases of anemia (determined by a quick blood test), a doctor will often advise an increase of iron in the diet. Iron is an essential mineral that enables the body to produce hemoglobin, the protein necessary to transport the oxygen. Even if a postpartum mom is not clinically anemic, a reduction in her iron supply may leave her feeling even more in need of a nap than she might otherwise feel. Red meat, chicken, and fish are good sources of iron. Vegetarians, fear not! Iron supply may be maintained by choosing dried beans, dried fruit, and leafy green vegetables like spinach or Swiss chard. Vitamin C supports the absorption of iron, so be sure to include foods like kiwi fruit, lemons, bell peppers, and berries as well.

Among its many unpleasant side-effects, sleep deprivation can also confuse the appetite, making it difficult to distinguish true hunger from the urge to eat. A lack of sleep can upset the hormones responsible for monitoring hunger and wakefulness, explains Gilroy. She offers one way to counteract this effect is to choose foods high in fiber, which are likely to increase the feeling of fullness (not to mention keep the colon happy) (pers. comm.).

MOOD

Got chocolate? If not, here is a good excuse to enjoy some. This delectable dessert comes with some mood-boosting side-effects, according to a recent article published in the journal *Nutrition Reviews* (Scholey and Owen 2013, 665–681). Incidentally, a number of these studies also suggest that chocolate improves cognitive functioning. Chocolate can have a positive effect on serotonin—the happy juice— in the brain and has been shown to enhance endorphin production just as exercise does. When looking for the sweet treat, choose a high quality dark chocolate with simple, natural ingredients. Some bars will indicate the percentage of cacao on the front of the label— that's a good sign. Since chocolate is not exactly low-calorie (if only), try and limit the serving size to the recommendation on the package if losing weight is on the agenda. One serving is often less than one whole bar. New moms who want to watch their weight should get into the habit of checking the serving size on labels. Also, consider using a serving of cocoa powder as an ingredient in smoothies or as an addition to a warm drink.

PHYSICAL HEALING

Food can either enable or disable healing in the months after birth. Regardless of whether you had a vaginal delivery or a C-section, the body needs time to recover. Replenishing the blood supply, mending tears or scars, and establishing a new hormonal equilibrium are tall tasks. Help the body along by choosing foods that provide healing benefits.

Protein is found in most living organisms. One of three macronutrients (carbohydrates and fats are the others), protein facilitates the growth of our muscles, tissues, and hair. Protein also keeps the immune system operating properly and helps us to feel full after a meal. It is easy to see why protein is a macronutrient—essential for life. Good sources of protein include meat, poultry, fish, and dairy. Vegetarians and vegans can find it in nuts and beans.

A small amount of zinc, an element found in nature, is also helpful in healing the body. Good sources of zinc include red meat and seafood. Decent vegetarian sources are pumpkin seeds, dark chocolate, garbanzo beans, and other legumes.

Vitamins, including C and A, will further enable postpartum repair. Vitamin C can be found in a variety of fruit and vegetables, while vitamin A is abundant in orange colored vegetables, like butternut squash, as well as dark and leafy veggies, like collard greens. If you find roughage a bit hard to choke down (you're not alone), consider including some in a blended fruit smoothie. Your body will be happy and so will your taste buds.

NURSING

Nursing moms have a few additional dietary considerations. The doctor or midwife may have already mentioned (hopefully) the need to consume some extra calories to ensure the body can produce milk. The average amount of supplemental calories required is five hundred per day, but everyone is different. Factors, including the size and appetite of your baby as well as your own size and activity level, may influence how many additional calories are appropriate. Use five hundred as a guideline and adjust accordingly depending on your doctor's recommendation and your energy level on a given day.

In the early postpartum period when baby is nursing every couple of hours, your milk supply is being replenished often. This means there is a higher demand for fluid (water is a great choice) and calories than there will be as baby grows older. A carbohydrate snack around half an hour before bedtime can help aid sleep and supply some calories for milk production during the night.

Some of my go-tos: two cups of air-popped popcorn mixed with a handful of raisins and a sprinkle of cinnamon (dee-lish!), a serving of whole-grain cereal with a cup of low-fat milk, or a slice of whole-wheat toast topped with a smear of nut butter and a few banana slices. (Unless you have a nut allergy, or there is a family history of nut allergies, the American Academy of Pediatrics reports it is safe to eat nut butter while breastfeeding.)

EATING IN THE REAL (MOM) WORLD

Even those who love to cook may just not find the time, energy, or satisfaction in the kitchen at this stage. If a spare half-hour pops up, a nap may be more enticing than making a meal. So, the question then becomes: How can food be used to your best advantage when you have minimal free time and even less energy? Here are some top tips and tricks to consider:

SNACK SMART

Keep nutritionally dense, tasty snacks on hand. Fruit, boiled eggs, cheese, and whole grain breads and crackers are good staples. Buy precut vegetables to save time and enjoy them with store bought hummus or nut butters.

"BUMP UP" A READY-MADE MEAL

Frozen dinners are not the enemy. Sometimes they are a saving grace. Boost the nutritional value by adding some whole foods to the meal such as pre-washed baby spinach, cherry tomatoes, or carrot sticks.

Wondering how to pick the best bets from the vast assortment in the freezer section? Check the ingredients on the package. Steer clear of those containing not-so-savory artificial sweeteners and preservatives. If you see names like butylated hydroxytoluene (BHT), sodium benzoate, or sodium nitrate/nitrite, keep your shopping cart moving! Same goes for partially hydrogenated oils and high fructose corn syrup. Review the nutrition info, too. Frozen dinners have a bad (but well-deserved) reputation when it comes to sugar (stick with less than 10g) and salt (keep it under 700mg). Amy's is a good brand to keep an eye out for, offering a tasty assortment of organic options.

MAKE THE MOST OF THE MOST IMPORTANT MEAL

Breakfast is the most important meal of the day, right? Maybe. Maybe not. A recent *New York Times* article points to a long history of flawed and biased research that calls into question the common philosophy (Carroll 2016). Whether or not breakfast reigns supreme, you deserve to start your day with a satisfying meal. Quick and tasty choices include a serving of Greek yogurt with a little granola and some berries, or a bowl of low-sugar cereal with milk.

PLAYING WITH PASTA

Many grocery stores now carry more than the typical dry, white pasta. Check out those made with a variety of grains such as quinoa or millet, or use these unprocessed grains in lieu of pasta or rice. They are just as easy to make as the traditional kind but will provide greater nutrition. Here are two scrumptious options courtesy of Patricia Gilroy:

Quinoa with roasted veggies & feta

Roast ½ a sliced red bell pepper, ½ a sliced green bell pepper, ½ a sliced red onion, and 2 whole, unpeeled cloves of garlic in a tablespoon of olive oil at 375°F (190°C) for 30 minutes. Remove the garlic and squeeze the soft pulp into the vegetables. In the same roasting pan, add ½ cup cooked quinoa and combine well to absorb the juices from veggies. Move to a plate and serve sprinkled with ¼ cup crumbled feta and 2–3 torn basil leaves.

Millet pilaf

Cook a cup of diced vegetables (onions, celery, carrots) with a clove of garlic in a tablespoon of olive oil until softened. Add ½ cup millet and cook for 1 minute while stirring. Add 1 cup of vegetable or chicken stock. Bring to a boil and reduce the heat to low. Cover and simmer for about 30 minutes until all of the liquid has been absorbed. Stir in ½ cup chopped parsley and a squeeze of lemon juice. Serve as a side dish for meat or fish, or add some beans for a full meal.

KEEP UP THE VITAMINS

If you took a prenatal vitamin throughout your pregnancy, continue to take it for at least six weeks through the postpartum period. Doing so will help to replenish much-needed nutrients.

FiNAL FOOD FOR THOUGHT

In early motherhood, good nutrition and a sound relationship with eating is important. But being gentle with oneself is equally, if not more, valuable. This is not the time to craft the perfect diet. It does not exist anyway. If you are breastfeeding, rest assured that breast milk is nutritionally adequate within a large range of dietary choices. Since weight loss never seems to be far from a new mother's mind, try to remember that while some women shed pounds within a few weeks, most of us do not. For those who want to lose the baby weight, there will be ample time to do so later on.

Concentrate now on incorporating some of these ideas into your daily life. Shift the focus away from calorie counting and more toward mindful, enjoyable eating. The meal guide that follows offers a mouth-watering way to put this knowledge into practice.

MEAL PLANNER GUIDE

This delectable and nutritionally sound weekly meal plan for new mamas comes courtesy of Nutritional Therapist (and dedicated mother of three) Patricia Gilroy. As you enjoy reviewing it, please remember that this is a time when food should be used as a health-enabler, not another stressor. Pick and choose what works for you and what whets your appetite.

MONDAY

BREAKFAST

Oatmeal Parfait

Overnight oats (made with 2% milk and a bit of maple syrup) topped with low-fat Greek yogurt and a sprinkle of blueberries

LUNCH

Turkey Salad Sandwich

Whole-grain roll with turkey breast, salad leaves, avocado, and tomato slices

DINNER

"Red" Salmon

Salmon steak baked with red bell peppers, red onions, and garlic

Sides: steamed broccoli; boiled baby potatoes with a bit of olive oil and lemon juice

SNACKS

1 hard-boiled egg; carrot and celery sticks with hummus for dipping

Individually wrapped cheese (e.g., Babybel, string cheese, etc.) with a portioned pack of whole-grain crackers

TIME-SAVING TRICKS

- Skip the stove and opt for overnight oats. Place a bowl in the fridge overnight and it'll be ready in the morning!
- Buy pre-washed salad greens.
- Consider using individually packaged frozen salmon steaks (wild-caught is preferable to farm-raised).
- Buy "steam in the bag" broccoli florets.
- Boil a bunch of eggs at the same time. In the shell, they may be stored in the fridge for up to a week.

HEALTHFUL TIPS

- Oats provide soluble fiber, which gives a longer-lasting feeling of fullness.
- Red peppers have vitamin C for healing and iron absorption.
- Broccoli has fiber, protein, and folate. (Folate levels may be low following pregnancy.)

TUESDAY

BREAKFAST

Bright-Eyed Morning Sandwich

Sliced hard-boiled egg & avocado on whole-wheat bread

LUNCH

Personalized Pasta Salad

Whole wheat pasta (served hot or cold) topped with a serving of low-fat mozzarella cheese; include any of the following no-cook additions: pesto, halved cherry tomatoes, olives, canned tuna, basil

Side

Mixed salad leaves dressed with a teaspoon of olive oil and a splash of balsamic vinegar

DINNER

Bite-Sized Beef Stir-Fry

Stir fry lean, bite-sized beef strips with vegetables (green beans or snap peas), garlic, and a little store-bought ginger puree or thin slices of fresh ginger. Add ½ cup of cashew nuts; season with soy sauce.

Side: brown or basmati rice

SNACKS

Toast with nut butter (almond, cashew, etc.), sliced banana, and grated dark chocolate

A serving of low-fat yogurt with a piece of fruit

DAYNA KURTZ | 71

TIME-SAVING TRICKS

- Use pre-cubed or pre-shredded low-fat mozzarella cheese.
- Use a frozen, stir-fry vegetable mix.
- Use minute rice or boil-in-bag.

HEALTHFUL TIPS

- Avocados are very high in folate and fiber, essential to postpartum well-being. They are also a generally nutritious food containing potassium, vitamin C, and vitamin E, as well as heart healthy fats.
- Low-fat mozzarella provides calcium for bone health.
- Lean beef contains protein, zinc, and iron, which will work to boost postpartum healing, immunity, and energy.
- Brown rice may help maintain energy levels.
- Basmati rice is a better option if iron levels are low, since brown rice may affect iron absorption.
- Cashews contain calcium, monounsaturated fatty acids, and magnesium. Low levels of magnesium may contribute to depressed mood and anxiety.

WEDNESDAY

BREAKFAST

Lite-Bite Toast

Whole-wheat toast with a scoop of low-fat ricotta cheese and "no added sugar" fruit spread

LUNCH

Savory Tomato Soup

Tomato soup with beans and whole-wheat or whole-grain crackers

DINNER

Classic Skillet Chicken

Brown cubed chicken in a skillet with a bit of olive oil. Toss in a tablespoon of flour seasoned with smoked paprika, cumin, salt, and black pepper. Add diced onion, celery, garlic, carrots, and peppers. Cook on low heat until onions are translucent. Add a can of tomatoes and a can of white beans. Continue to cook over a low heat for about 40 minutes.

Sides: baked potato or brown rice; mixed greens

SNACKS

2 cups of air-popped popcorn mixed with a handful of raisins and sprinkle of cinnamon

Small bowl of low-sugar cereal with a serving of low-fat milk

TIME-SAVING TRICKS

- Use a freshly made (i.e., not from a can) store-bought organic soup.
- Use a package of taco seasoning mix instead of mixing individual spices.
- Dinner leftovers can be baked in the oven with a topping of breadcrumbs and cheese, or mixed with some rice and cheese in a burrito.

HEALTHFUL TIPS

- Chicken has protein for healing and satiety, and magnesium for mood enhancement.
- Beans also contain protein, iron, magnesium, and fiber for regularity, as well as folate, which is often in need of replenishment after pregnancy.
- Baked potatoes are filling and have potassium, which can lower blood pressure. Potato skins have fiber and vitamin C.

THURSDAY

BREAKFAST

Simple Scramble

Two scrambled eggs with tomato slices and a serving of low-fat cheddar cheese

LUNCH

"Throw It In" Noodles

Rice noodles or whole-wheat angel hair pasta tossed with a touch of sesame or walnut oil (to prevent sticking). Toss with a few avocado slices and any of the following add-ins: ¾ cup of shelled edamame OR 3 ounces of chicken or salmon or cubed tofu. Add any of the following: chopped scallions, diced cucumber, mixed salad leaves, halved cherry tomatoes, handful of fresh cilantro, and/or handful of fresh mint. *Dressing: 1 tablespoon toasted sesame oil; 1 teaspoon soy sauce; 1 tablespoon of rice vinegar, white wine vinegar, or lime juice; and 1 teaspoon of tomato ketchup. Place all in a small jar and shake well.*

DINNER

"Good Ole" Meatballs and Spaghetti, Made Better

Use frozen store-bought turkey meatballs and a sauce made from half store-bought pasta sauce and half canned tomato puree, mixed together. Add a variety of fresh vegetables to the sauce (diced tomatoes, onions, peppers, cooked zucchini, or eggplant) and serve with whole-wheat spaghetti or other pasta.

Side: green salad

SNACKS

A cup of sliced strawberries with a scoop of low-fat ricotta cheese
Fruit & nut bar (e.g., Kind bar) with a glass of low-fat milk

TIME-SAVING TRICKS

- Scrambled eggs can be made in the microwave for speed and to save on dishwashing.
- With the noodles, use leftover chicken from the night before.
- Tofu can usually be eaten straight from the package (check directions) or easily baked and kept in the fridge for 2–3 days.
- Dressing may be made in larger quantities and stored in the fridge.

HEALTHFUL TIPS

- Strawberries are a great source of vitamin C, while low-fat ricotta cheese provides calcium and protein.
- Edamame is a good vegetarian source of protein. Baked tofu also provides protein and magnesium.
- This quick dinner is a well-balanced meal containing, protein, carbohydrates, fiber, and a little fat.
- It is important to balance out the frozen and jarred foods (which will most likely be high in sodium) with some fresh fruit and vegetables.

FRIDAY

BREAKFAST

Sensational Smoothies

Choose any one of the following:

Tropical: 1 cup chopped mango, fresh or frozen, ½ cup silken tofu, and 1 cup coconut milk

Oat cookie: ½ cup of oats, 1 very ripe banana, 1 cup of milk, ½ teaspoon cinnamon, and 1 tablespoon of peanut butter

Green: ½ a ripe avocado, handful of baby spinach leaves, 1 green apple, a slice of fresh ginger, and 1 cup of diced melon (cantaloupe or honeydew)

PB&J: ½ cup of oats, 1 cup of milk, ½ cup of frozen mixed berries, 1 tablespoon of peanut butter, and 1 teaspoon of honey

LUNCH

Choice Chicken Sandwich

1 slice of whole-wheat bread topped with 2 ounces chicken breast slices, 1 ounce low-fat cheese, lettuce, tomato, onion, and mustard

DINNER

Baked Chicken & Nightshades

Combine chicken thighs; cubes of zucchini, eggplant, and sweet potato; and chunks of red bell pepper with some avocado oil, crushed garlic, lemon juice, salt, and pepper in a baking tray. Bake in a preheated oven at 400°F (204°C) for approximately 40 minutes, checking frequently.

SNACKS

Handful of any combination of nuts and dried fruit

Serving of yogurt with a piece of fruit

TIME-SAVING TRICKS

- An easy-to-clean smoothie maker can do double-duty to puree baby food.
- Buy packages of pre-sliced, frozen fruit and store in the freezer.
- Smoothies are a great choice when nursing or bottle-feeding.

HEALTHFUL TIPS

- Add a handful of baby spinach to any of the smoothies for added folate and fiber. This will likely not affect the taste, but will provide a health boost!
- All nuts are nutritionally dense, containing protein and monounsaturated fats. (Walnuts are a particularly good source of omega-3 fats.) They are rich in B-vitamins, including folate—which can become depleted in pregnancy—vitamin E, and minerals such as iron, calcium, zinc, and selenium. Notably they are rich in magnesium. Low magnesium levels have been linked to postpartum depression, as well as general anxiety, tension, and depression (Etebary et al., 2010).
- While chicken thighs are higher in calories and fat than chicken breasts, they work better in this dish because they can be baked without drying out. They also contain higher levels of zinc and B-vitamins than white-meat chicken.

SATURDAY

BREAKFAST

Mashed Cherry Toast

1 slice of whole-wheat toast with mashed avocado (mash the avocado until it becomes like a dip) and cherry tomatoes.

LUNCH

Fish 'n' Beans

½ can of mixed beans with a serving of canned tuna in water. Serve with a side of cucumber and leafy greens and dressing of olive oil, vinegar, and splash of Tabasco or other hot sauce. Serve with a whole-wheat tortilla or a serving of low-salt blue-corn tortilla chips.

DINNER

"Nutty" Kale & Pasta

Lightly toast some walnuts and set aside. Sauté some frozen kale with some crushed garlic, mix in the walnuts, and stir into the pasta; drizzle with olive oil and top with a little shave of Parmesan and a squeeze of lemon juice. Be sure to make extra for lunch tomorrow!

SNACKS

1 ½ ounces of reduced-fat cheddar cheese with apple slices
Small bowl of low-sugar cereal with a serving of low-fat milk

HEALTHFUL TIPS

- Beans provide magnesium, fiber, and protein.
- Tuna contains omega-3 fatty acids, including DHA.
- Apples are a good source of vitamin C, and cheese provides protein.
- Kale is high in folate and vitamin C.
- Walnuts provide omega-3 fats and magnesium.

SUNDAY

BREAKFAST

Sweet & Savory Oatmeal

Oatmeal with one or more of the following toss-ins: a dollop of almond butter, a sprinkle of sunflower or sesame seeds, toasted coconut flakes, sliced bananas, blueberries, or raisins
A glass of low-fat milk

LUNCH

"Nutty" Kale & Pasta Redux

Leftover kale pasta salad from last night's dinner

DINNER

Crock-Pot Mexican Chicken

Combine 1 can of beans (black, pinto, or kidney) with 1 can of crushed tomatoes and 1 packet of taco seasoning. Place 3–4 skinless, boneless chicken breasts on top. Bake 3–4 hours on high or 8–10 on low. Sprinkle with low-fat cheddar cheese before serving.

Side: brown rice

SNACKS

½ a mashed avocado (mash the avocado until it becomes like a dip) with rice crackers and vegetable sticks
Individually wrapped cheese (e.g., Babybel, string cheese, etc.) with a portioned pack of whole-grain crackers

TIME-SAVING TRICKS

- Buy pre-cut vegetables for dipping, often available in the produce aisle.
- A Crock-Pot is a super-useful appliance in the post-partum period (and beyond) because it is time-efficient and allows for food to be made in large quantities (for leftovers). Consider buying Crock-Pot liners to make clean-up a snap!
- Use minute-rice if time is short.

HEALTHFUL TIPS

- Nut butters and seeds are good sources of protein, calcium, and healthy fats.
- Raisins are a good source of iron (essential for restoring blood supply postpartum) and fiber (needed to keep digestion running smoothly.)

FLEXERCISE

HOW A LITTLE WORKOUT CAN GO A LONG WAY

Take care of your body. It's the only place you have to live.

—Jim Rohn, American entrepreneur

I mages in the media are filled with celebrity moms who are back to size zero seemingly moments after giving birth. What we do not see are photos of their staff (personal chefs, trainers, nannies, housekeepers, etc.) who are available to them around the clock helping them to regain their skinny status. Most women do not have the resources to drop the baby weight in an instant, but the societal expectation and the judgment remain.

What if, as new mothers, we reframe how we think about exercise? Whether someone was a gym rat before pregnancy or considered running to the ladies' room to be a complete workout,

A little workout can offer some pretty big gains beyond weight loss.

transitioning to motherhood brings with it an invaluable opportunity to consider our thoughts and feelings about fitness in life. Sporting the skinnies again is a fine motivation, but there are many more reasons to include exercise at this particular stage in time. It may come as a pleasant surprise that even a little workout can offer some pretty big gains beyond weight loss.

A *Forbes* magazine article listed the number-one reason people give for not working out is lack of time (Dusen 2008, par. 3). If time was sparse before your baby, chances are it is even harder to come by now. Happily, the exercises described later in this chapter will prove that a good workout does not require a big time commitment. What it does require is creativity and flexibility, and not just the physical kind.

WHY FLEXERCISE?

Welcome to a new way to think about working out—a more mother-friendly way. Forget exercise. Embrace *flexercise*. Flexercise is about reflecting on the motivation for fitness at this particular time and then being purposeful in choosing how to incorporate it into new-mom-life. As a parent, preserving physical and emotional health becomes even more meaningful. Learning to flexercise makes it possible to do both. Just how to do it will be explored a bit later in the chapter, but, generally, the flexercise philosophy offers that a workout should:

- make you feel better, not worse
- fit comfortably into your daily (or nightly) routine
- be adaptable to your current level of fitness
- include a modification to be done with or without your baby

- embrace the reality that sometimes rest is more important than motion

Embrace the reality that sometimes rest is more important than motion.

We'll take a look at how flexercise can work in the real world of mothering in a moment. First though, here's a quick look at why a workout is worth doing in the midst of the bleary-eyed, postpartum haze.

YOUR MENTAL HEALTH

The positive correlation between exercise and mood enhancement is well researched. Natural endorphins released during exercise, the ones that make us feel good, are not unlike those brain chemicals stimulated by antidepressant medications but without any unpleasant side effects.

Beyond the endorphin rush, the emotional lift provided by exercise is also likely to give a new mom a bump in her self-esteem, according to a study in *Health Care for Women International* (Currie and Develin 2002, 882–93). It is no secret that the formula for weight loss is more calories burned off than taken in through food. Exercise expends calories. The more one moves, the more calories come off. The result is likely to be a noticeably slimmer waistline. For moms who are eager to lose the baby weight, this measure of progress toward the goal is bound to give a boost to both the ego and the mood.

YOUR SENSE OF SELF

Noted Stanford University psychologist Albert Bandura is credited with developing the concept of self-efficacy. Broadly defined, self-efficacy is a series of beliefs someone has about her ability to do certain things. These beliefs influence action, behavior, choices, and how individuals think and feel. For example, my self-efficacy around public speaking is pretty good. Put me in front of a crowd and I feel right at home. I can communicate clearly and in an engaging manner. I'm in my element. By contrast, my self-efficacy when it comes to calculus hovers somewhere around non-existent. Put me at a desk with a problem to solve and I'm sunk in a matter of seconds.

Becoming a mother has a profound impact on self-efficacy in many different domains, affecting both a woman's psychological well-being, as well as her child's social and emotional development (Shorey, Chan, Seng-Chong, and Hong-Gu 2015, 1604–22). There is a direct relationship between self-efficacy and exercise. Postpartum women who engaged in a strength-based training program were found to have greater self-efficacy around exercise than postpartum women who did not, a 2014 study revealed (LeCheminant et al., 414–21). In other words, those who *believed* in their ability to exercise more, exercised more.

Personal fitness trainer and educator Doug Jackson offers that a stronger belief in one's ability to work out is associated with better adherence to an exercise routine, higher overall fitness levels, and a greater likelihood of achieving personal fitness goals like losing weight or completing a first 5K race. Even a short bout of moderate exercise has been found to increase self-efficacy. As few as ten minutes of aerobic exercise was enough to increase beliefs in one's exercise capabilities and enhance emotional well-being (David and Butki 1998, 268–80). A little really does go a long way!

YOUR MILK

Some women "express" concern about the effect of exercise on their milk—both the ability to produce it and the way it tastes to their babies. Lactic acid, a natural compound made in the body during exercise, can be detected in breast milk following exercise.

However, the bulk of current research indicates that for postpartum women who exercise in a mild to moderate capacity, the lactic acid has no impact on either production or baby's preference for it. If your baby seems fussy during a post-workout feeding, consider fitting in a feeding before you exercise. This will not only make the work out more comfortable (imagine holding a plank position with a full bosom—yikes!), but will also allow more time for the lactic acid levels in the breast milk to dissipate before feeding again.

YOUR BONES

Bone density can actually be lost during breastfeeding! Most of us are never told this vital piece of health information. Calcium, used to make milk, is extracted from the bones, resulting in a certain amount of bone loss. For many, bone mass is restored after lactation stops. But this is not the case for all. The good news is that studies demonstrate both aerobic and strength training exercises may help to reduce the rate of bone loss throughout the time period mothers are nursing (Lovelady et al. 2009, 1902–07).

YOUR HEART

The American Heart Association and World Heart Federation cite cardiovascular disease, which includes heart disease and stroke, as the number one killer of women around the world. According to a number of studies in the last few years, mothers diagnosed with complications, such as preeclampsia and gestational diabetes, during pregnancy are at increased risk for cardiovascular disease later in life. This underscores the therapeutic necessity of incorporating moderate exercise to improve and maintain good heart health. A group of postnatal women engaged in an exercise program demonstrated improvements in haemodynamic function (the flow of blood) and a reduction in blood pressure, both of which reduce the risk of heart disease (Carpenter et al. 2015, 1–15). Your heart beats for you around the clock. Make her job a little easier by exercising to keep her going strong.

YOUR SLEEP

Postpartum fatigue can be brutal. Brutal! (My son is eight and sometimes I feel I'm still trying to catch up on the sleep I missed out on!) Most new moms are unable to avoid it at least during the first few months and often beyond that. Exercise is one simple and effective remedy that can help mitigate the effects of sleep deprivation, according to a compelling study published in the *Annals of Behavioral Medicine*. The research found that a home-based, individual aerobic exercise program reduced fatigue, both physical and mental, in women with postpartum depression (Dritsa et al. 2008, 179–87). Another team of researchers found that a group of postnatal women who practiced in-home Pilates, a method of exercise designed to enhance strength, flexibility, posture, and awareness, had lower levels of physical and mental fatigue than their non-practicing peers (Ashrafinia et al. 2015, 169–73).

YOUR SOCIAL LIFE

Yes! You can still have a social life after having a baby. In fact, one of the beautiful aspects of exercise is that it can offer a time for quiet introspection or social engagement. As a new mom, opportunities for both are so important. Many areas offer group exercise classes for new mothers. Check out the Resources section in the back of the book to find

One of the beautiful aspects of exercise is that it can offer a time for quiet introspection or social engagement.

a local class. Some gyms also include group classes or have on-site babysitting so you can workout while your baby plays. Call the local gym to find out what is available. Don't want to be beholden to a class schedule?

Any activity that elevates the heart rate and/or strengthens the muscles and bones has value.

Grab the stroller and a friend and head out for a walk together.

We've explored some pretty compelling reasons to get moving, though starting a routine is often the hardest part. If your motivation is lacking, remember this: *any* activity that elevates your heart rate and/or strengthens your muscles and bones has value. Traditional exercise falls into two categories: cardiovascular or aerobic, and strength or resistance. Cardiovascular exercises are those that elevate the heart rate. The benefits of aerobics are numerous, ranging from improving heart health, lowering blood pressure, losing and maintaining weight, and enhancing psychological well-being. Resistance-training activities are intended to build the strength, endurance, and sometimes the size of muscles. The American College of Sports Medicine reports that strength-training can decrease the risk of osteoporosis, combat sarcopenia (the loss of lean muscle mass as people age), and lower body fat (ACSM 2013). Most reputable US health organizations recommend a combination of both aerobic and resistance exercises. The Center for Disease Control suggests about two-and-a-half hours of moderate cardiovascular exercise over the course of the week (for example, a brisk thirty-minute walk Monday through Friday) and two days of resistance training targeting the major muscle groups (CDC 2008). Within these guidelines, there is ample opportunity for flexercise. The kinds of activities and the ways they can be included day-to-day are varied.

PRE-FLEXERCISE CHECKLIST

Medical clearance. Prior to beginning any exercise program, everyone (mom or not) needs to be sure she is healthy enough to workout. Particularly in the postpartum stage, make sure to have the doctor's okay.

A word on water. Drink up! Noted pediatrician William Sears recommends that nursing mothers should aim to drink eight ounces of water with each feeding, usually eight to ten times daily (2017). Nursing or not, be sure to keep water close during a workout and take breaks to sip slowly.

Dress for success. Help the "girls" by wearing a bra with solid support. Breasts feeling especially full? Consider wearing two. Choose an athletic pant that provides a good foundation for the abdominal region and pelvis. Your breathing should not be restricted, but a comfortable, structured lift will help ensure your comfort while moving. Don't underestimate the power of your workout wear; your wardrobe can have a powerful impact on how you feel.

Nurse? Then nurse first. Pumping or feeding before working out will make both you and your baby happier. Expressing milk in advance will make your breasts feel lighter. For the very small number of babies who do notice a taste-change in mom's milk following an intense workout, they, too, will be happy for a pre-workout meal.

Grab a simple snack. Be sure to have a light snack half an hour or so beforehand. Working out on an empty stomach can leave you feeling like you have morning sickness all over again.

Be body conscious. If something does not feel good, and certainly if it is painful, stop! This is not the time to attempt an Olympic trial or go for a new personal record. The human body is a wonderful barometer of knowing how much is too much. Trust it.

> Embrace the new flexercise practice: do what can be done now, with minimal effort or planning.

Embrace the new flexercise practice: do what can be done now, with minimal effort or planning. A workout should bolster well-being, not deplete it. Whether you manage five minutes or a full hour, give yourself credit where credit is due. Focus on what you accomplished in that particular workout. Much like the act of mothering itself, exercise almost always presents another opportunity to try again tomorrow.

GO FLEXERCISE!

CARDIOVASCULAR EXERCISE

Aerobic, or cardiovascular exercise, is any form of movement that elevates the heart rate. One of the best forms is the one many babies learn around their first birthdays: walking.

THE WONDER OF A WALK AROUND THE BLOCK: JENNIFER'S STORY

I had a tremendously upsetting experience in labor. My hope was to have a natural childbirth, but after sixteen hours of contractions and very little progress, I was exhausted and felt pressured to have a C-section. When I brought Catherine home, I just felt so low. All I wanted was to be able to relax and snuggle with her, but I was in so much discomfort. My sister also had a C-section with her son about a year before. She told me that her daily afternoon walk saved her in the first weeks after my nephew was born. A walk around the block didn't seem like a wonder-drug, but I figured I would give it a try.

*One week after I gave birth, I wrapped Catherine up in the stroller
and we headed outside for about twenty minutes. We stayed close
to home and kept a leisurely pace. I was surprised by how much
I enjoyed it! I don't know if it was the fresh air or just being out-
doors, but I felt so revived when we came back home. I was more
energized and less bothered by the lingering abdominal pain. Our
afternoon walks together became a daily part of the routine that we
both looked forward to.*

Walking is among the best forms of exercise—especially in the pre-
through postpartum stages—and offers numerous advantages.

Walking

- is one of the safest aerobic exercises for most people
- requires no equipment (other than sneakers or comfortable shoes)
- may be done at no cost
- may be done almost anywhere
- can be adjusted to your current fitness level
- may be done alone or in a social group
- is virtually free of negative side-effects
- is relatively easy on the joints and ligaments (often tender
  following pregnancy)
- is a scientifically proven treatment in reducing postpartum depression

A group of mothers, all of whom had given birth within the year
and were suffering from postpartum depression, were recruited to
participate in a study on walking as a therapeutic tool. The women
were divided into two groups. One group met for walking sessions, three times a week for a period of twelve weeks. The other
group did not engage in organized walking. At the halfway point,

the walkers had significantly reduced depressive symptoms as compared to those in the control group. Not only did the depression continue to subside through the end of the program, but the moms who moved also demonstrated notable improvement in aerobic fitness as compared to their peers who did not (Currie and Develin 2002, 882–93). Not bad for a walk around the block.

Still not moved by the idea of walking? Consider this: Some 20 percent of Americans suffer from either Seasonal Affective Disorder (SAD) or a less severe variation of winter blues (Targum and Rosenthal 2008, 31–33). Moms who deliver in the fall or winter may have the added challenge of combatting the commonly depressive effects of shorter, darker days. Going for a walk provides an opportunity to be outside and get a dose of feel-good natural light and vitamin D—precious commodities during the winter months. The sunlight exposure may not be sufficient on its own to combat SAD or the blues, but it can help, especially in combination with the aerobic benefit of a walk.

Another advantage of a walk outside is the opportunity to resume contact with the world beyond the walls of the nursery. In the early days and weeks of baby care, forgetting that there is a community larger than you and your baby is easy to do. Simply stepping out into that environment again can help reestablish a sense of connection with other (grown-up) people.

So how can you weave walking into your mom-life? Here are some simple suggestions:

Ditch the car. Grab the stroller and walk to the local dry cleaners, grocery store, post office, or library. If the stroller does not have ample storage, consider bringing a backpack for items that will be dropped off or picked up along the way.

Make steps matter. Use a pedometer to keep track of how many steps are logged or download the Charity Miles app on a smart phone. This free app not only tracks your mileage, but, through corporate sponsorship, allows the user to earn cash for a favorite charity with each and every step. At the end of an exercise session, take pride in the knowledge that your workout was for a good cause.

Don't wait for fair weather. Turn the shopping mall into a walking mall. Spend calories instead of cash.

Hop on/hop off. If you regularly use public transportation, consider getting off the bus or subway one or two stops early and walking part of the way to your final destination.

Gather together. Join (or start) a stroller-walking group in your local community. A group walk offers the added benefit of socializing with other grown-ups. Or, call up a friend (new mom or not) and ask if she would be up for a walk together.

If walking does not feel like the right speed, there are many other aerobic activities to get your heart pumping. Whether these exercises are done alone or in a group setting, running, cycling, and swimming all offer excellent benefits for cardiovascular and psychological health. Here is a little information on each, keeping your new-mom status in mind.

Running

Women who were runners before their babies were born may find themselves missing that addictive runner's high. Running can be an excellent way to lose the excess baby weight and begin to look and feel like oneself again. But, before lacing up your sneakers, be mindful. During pregnancy, ligaments, the cartilage that connects one bone to another and holds joints together, become more flexible. Relaxin, the hormone responsible for the increased malleability, while highly useful in helping your body grow and deliver a baby, can also make a mom less sturdy. As relaxin levels decrease, ligaments and joints will become firmer; this can take a period of some months to occur. In the interim, take it slow to reduce the risk of strain or injury. Listen to your body—it usually knows.

When you're feeling run-ready again, make sure to start out slowly and increase your pace gradually over a period of months. Stick to a well-known course and consider running with a partner for both companionship and safety. Though an investment, a jogging stroller specially designed for the purpose of running or jogging may be worthwhile. Be sure to check the infant height and weight requirements before use. And if you do run with your baby, be prepared to stop for a diaper change or dropped pacifier. Running with your little one can be wonderful, but it is a different experience than running on your own. If you set your expectations accordingly (whether heading out for a run or any other activity), you are more likely to enjoy the course.

Cycling

Like running, cycling is a wonderful exercise to promote weight loss and maintain a strong, healthy heart. And cycling can be easier on the joints than running since it does not involve any pounding. Riding a bike presents its own considerations. If soreness or discomfort from a vaginal birth is an issue, and certainly if bleeding or spotting are present, skip the bike entirely. Any irritation or aggravation to the area will not only be uncomfortable but may hinder the healing process. When you're ready to ride again, consider a stationary bike with a recumbent seat which may offer more comfort than a traditional bike seat. A bouncer can be placed next to a stationary bike so baby can watch you ride. While a thirty-minute cycle may not be possible, something is better than nothing. Riding outside? Please put on a helmet! A bad hair day is nothing compared to a head injury. (I'm always amazed by the number of parents I see who carefully place helmets on their kiddos, but leave their own heads helmet-free. Taking steps to preserve your own safety is part of responsible parenting.) Most child bike seats or trailers have specific age, height, and weight requirements. Your baby should have solid head and neck control (usually established by about twelve months), so outdoor cycling may be a better option if and when childcare is available or as your baby grows into toddlerhood. If in doubt, check in with your pediatrician.

Swimming

If you are lucky enough to have access to a pool, swimming is the way to move. Swimming, like cycling, is a low impact sport, meaning it does not place additional stress on the joints, and it can be practiced through pregnancy and beyond. In addition, swimming works the entire body—upper, lower, and core—providing a real bang for your buck. Chlorine can be an irritant. If you had an episiotomy or vaginal tearing during birth or if there is residual vaginal discharge, hold off before diving in.

Swimming works the entire body—upper, lower, and core—providing a real bang for your buck.

Other types of cardio

The StairMasters, treadmills, ellipticals, and rowing machines found at most gyms are also designed for an aerobic workout. Some gyms now offer babysitting on-site. Ask about the options. Want to keep the cost down? Consider recruiting a mom-friend for a tag-team workout. One of you can provide childcare while the other gets her workout in, then switch.

Whichever cardiovascular activity you choose, be sure to finish it with five to ten minutes of a cool-down period. A leisurely walk is usually the easiest, along with some simple stretching. This will allow the heart-rate to come down and breathing to resume a normal pace. When I remember to do it, I like to offer up a sense of gratitude during my cool down. I may thank my body for the work she did, or acknowledge the privilege of being in nature, or express my gratitude for the conversation I enjoyed with a friend. Give it a try. You may find that it adds a layer of meaning to your experience.

STRENGTH TRAINING

When folks talk about baby weight, they usually mean the pounds put on in pregnancy. But after birth, the term can take on an entirely new meaning; we can use it to refer to the weight of your baby—which may be increasing quickly and dramatically! Lifting a newborn is a lot less taxing than lifting a six-month-old. Keeping bones and muscles strong and healthy will help not only in the tasks of day-to-day mothering, but also in looking and feeling better while you're doing them.

The American College of Sports Medicine defines strength or resistance training as "a form of physical activity that is designed to improve muscular fitness by exercising a muscle or group of muscles against external resistance" (2013). Resistance training aims to strengthen the major muscle groups of the body and provides a unique opportunity to be creative and fun in approaching fitness.

FINDING STRENGTH: MALLORY'S STORY

I hate the gym—always have. I joined one once and felt so self-conscious working out with other people around that I never went. When my son Brian was an infant, he wanted to be held all the time. I was okay holding him the first few months, but he was off the charts for height and weight—my husband is 6'7". By the time he was four months old, lifting him up was getting harder. I knew he was only going to get heavier and that I better do something if I wanted to have any hope of carrying him past his first birthday. So, two days a week I started a baby-and-me strength-training program. Much to my surprise, I liked it! A personal trainer came to my home and took me through a series of resistance training exercises. And the best part? She showed me how to use Brian in the exercises—he was my weight! Brian loved working out with me. The sessions gave us a different way to connect and bond with each other. And even though I think Brian thought it was just play time, I liked the idea that maybe he was seeing how strong his mommy could be, and that made me feel good.

Mallory discovered one of the special aspects of resistance training—the option to work out with your baby. Amidst the feeding, diaper changing, and tummy time, mommy/baby muscle-building can provide a welcome change of pace and welcome results, too. Even so, some moms may find that exercise time is somewhat sacred—just for them. They may prefer to spend their workouts either alone or in a class setting with other grown-ups. Sometimes it simply depends on the day and what child-care options are available or not. Bottom line: the workout that works best for *you* is the best workout.

The workout that works best for *you* is the best workout.

As a general guideline, the American College of Sports Medicine recommends some form of resistance training twice a week (2011, par. 6). Most fitness professionals are not transitioning to motherhood. Do what you can for the time being and give yourself credit. That is part of what flexercising is all about. Be open to the possibilities and make them work in the best way possible.

In addition to the physical and psychological benefits strength-training affords new mothers, the exercises outlined below provide additional advantages, including the ability to:

- make modifications depending on one's current fitness level
- choose variations on how to include baby or not
- use body weight for resistance, thereby eliminating the need for equipment
- perform many exercises almost anywhere

Strength-training preparation should include:

- selecting a space that is clear of baby toys and equipment and big enough for a yoga mat or large towel
- having water nearby
- bringing baby or something along that can be used for weight (free weights, hardcover books, two full water bottles, etc.)
- warming up muscles to reduce the risk of injury
- engaging your core by drawing in the navel to the spine at the start of each exercise; doing so will help to keep the abdominal muscles active

- exhaling on the hard part of each exercise (for example, when doing a push-up, inhale while coming down and exhale while pushing up)

These exercises are best performed when the muscles are warm and limber. Start out with a brief warm-up: five minutes of brisk walking around the home, going up and down the stairs, jumping jacks, jogging in place, or another activity that literally creates a warm feeling or even a little sweat. These exercises could even be performed after a hot bath or shower, as muscles will be more pliable.

Two varieties of strength-training exercises for each region of the body (upper, lower, and core) are detailed below. Video demonstrations of select exercises may be found by visiting dayna mkurtz.com.

LOWER BODY

Sumo squat

Why to do it: This is a terrific exercise for strengthening the muscles in the back and pelvis, the legs and butt, and, with a simple modification, the arms as well. Sumos are a great strength-building exercise to prepare for lifting your baby as she grows.

How to do it: Adopt a neutral stance on the mat. Your feet should be a little more than shoulder-width apart and your toes pointed out at about a 45-degree angle. Tuck the tailbone under to engage the abdominal muscles (when the muscles in the belly area contract they should feel tighter, as if they are "awake"). With your arms comfortably at either side, take a deep breath and slowly lower down by bending your knees. Be mindful that the knees remain in alignment over the toes and the upper body remains vertical. Exhale while slowly rising back to the original position. Aim for eight to ten repetitions.

How to do it with baby: To include your little one, hold him by placing one arm under his bottom and the other around his waist. He may be either facing you or facing out. Hold him comfortably and firmly while squatting down and rising back up. Adding baby weight or a free weight, such as a heavy book or five-pound dumbbell, will provide a strengthening boost for the arms as well.

How to modify it: To make the sumo squat harder, either increase the number of repetitions to twelve to fifteen or add more weight. Want it easier? Shoot for five to seven repetitions or skip the weight altogether and let your arms rest by the sides of your body, or lightly rest them on a chair or table for greater stability.

Forward lunge

Why to do it: A lunge is also a great option for strengthening the leg muscles, including the quadriceps, hamstrings, calves, and the glutes. Like the sumo squat, a forward lunge offers a simple modification to incorporate some upper body work as well.

How to do it: From a standing position, draw the navel into the spine to engage the core abdominal muscles. With your hands on your hips, lift one foot and take a big step forward. As the forward foot lands, bend your back knee so that it gently brushes the ground and your front knee makes a 90-degree angle. The front knee should not go beyond the big toe. The upper body should remain upright. Remember to breathe, exhaling while lunging forward and inhaling while returning to a standing position. Aim for eight to ten repetitions.

How to do it with baby: Turn your baby so she is facing out and hold her comfortably with one arm supporting her bottom and the other arm around the waist. Hold her slightly in front of your body. While lunging forward, your baby should remain level. Be mindful to keep your shoulders nice and relaxed throughout.

How to modify it: To make the forward lunge harder, either increase the repetitions or the weight. To make it easier, skip the weight and place your hands on your hips, or hold a chair or table for added support.

UPPER BODY

Push-up

Why to do it: Before poo-pooing the push-up, here is why it is worth giving it a second thought. The push-up is easily modified based on fitness level and provides an excellent way to tone the chest, arms, and shoulder muscles. As a bonus, the push-up will also require the use of the rectus abdominis (the six-pack), other abdominal muscles, and the front thigh muscles (quadriceps). On busy days, the push-up is a great way to get a lot of strength training in in a little bit of time.

How to do it: The basic push-up is a fairly challenging exercise (for me, anyway). Depending on your current fitness level or feeling on a given day, use the modification provided. Begin by coming onto your hands and knees. (If you have any knee issues, use a hand towel or pillow underneath your knees for added cushion.) The hands may be slightly further than shoulder-width apart. Check that elbows are firm but not locked in place. Knees should be aligned with hips. Extend one leg out and then the other so that the feet are flexed with your toes curled underneath, making contact with the mat. You should now be in a plank position. Inhale while slowly lowering yourself down toward the mat, keeping the body straight from head to tailbone, and then exhale coming back up to the plank position. Aim for five to seven reps.

How to do it with baby: Moms and babies alike enjoy doing push-ups together. Place baby on his back on the mat. Come onto all fours so that he is equidistant between your hands. The push-up provides an ideal opportunity for nose-to-nose kisses!

How to modify it: To make the push-up harder, increase the repetitions and shoot for ten to twelve. To make it easier, from all fours, bring the knees closer together and bend them, so that your feet may be raised in the air and comfortably crossed at your ankles. Keep a straight line from the head to the tailbone while coming down and up.

Press-up

Why to do it: Want to be able to lift and carry your baby more easily and look good doing it? A press-up is a great exercise to choose. A strength builder for the biceps, triceps, often-neglected wrists, and some of the shoulder and chest musculature, the press-up is typically easier to do than the push-up because the body is largely supported.

How to do it: Begin by lying on your back with your knees bent and your feet flat on the floor. Tilt the pelvis so that the small of the back is flush with the mat. Doing so will engage your abdominal muscles. Grab your weights—a water bottle, book, or dumbbell in each hand—and exhale while pushing the weight straight up toward the ceiling. Try and keep your shoulders down. Slowly inhale while bringing the weight back down toward the chest. Aim for ten to twelve reps.

How to do it with baby: From the starting position, hold your baby face down on your chest with your hands under her armpits. Lift her slowly up, making sure her torso is strongly supported, then bring her back to your chest.

How to modify it: Go for fifteen reps to increase the difficulty level. To make it easier, use a lighter weight or keep the weight and stop at five to eight reps.

CORE

These days, the term "core" is used a lot in exercise lingo. When used here, it refers to the muscles in the front and back of the entire torso and pelvic region. These muscles are integral to supporting and maintaining the functionality of the whole body. Apart from the brain, all the major internal organs are located in the same region where the core musculature is located.

The core muscles undergo a shift during the pre- through postpartum phases. In pregnancy, the abdominal muscles serve to protect and house the baby and support the spine. During labor, abdominal muscles help to regulate breathing and assist the uterus in contracting to push the baby out. In the postpartum period, the abdominal muscles are often in need of toning to resume functioning as they did prior to pregnancy. Weak core muscles can lead to lower-back pain and can make the physical work of mothering, like lifting and carrying baby, more difficult.

Before engaging in strength training specifically aimed at working the abdominal muscles, take steps to ensure that these exercises may be engaged in safely, and that they will be of benefit not harm. First, perform a quick and easy assessment to check for diastasis recti. Diastasis recti is a separation of the rectus abdominis, the six-pack muscles on the left and right side of the belly. Diastasis recti is very common in pregnancy and the postpartum period, affecting as many as 50 to 60 percent of women. Usually there is no formal treatment required, as the rectus abdominis muscles may repair themselves.

Weak core muscles can lead to low-back pain and can make the physical work of mothering, like lifting and carrying baby, more difficult.

Determining the presence of a diastasis recti is easy by performing a simple self-exam. Begin by lying on the back on a flat surface with your knees bent and the soles of your feet on the floor. Place one hand behind your head. Slowly exhale while lifting the head and neck slightly off the ground as if performing a crunch. There should be a natural depression or gap about two inches above the navel, in the middle of the belly. With your other hand, see how many fingers are able to fit into the gap. Typically, one or two fingers may either dip slightly into the area or not move at all. If three or more fingers fit, or if the fingers bulge out instead, this is an indication of a possible separation of the rectus abdominis muscles. This is not cause for alarm. Consult with your ob-gyn, midwife, or a physical therapist to determine the severity of the separation and whether or not formal treatment is recommended.

Plank

Why to do it: Planks are a three *s*'s exercise: straightforward, simply-modified, and super-efficient. They are straightforward in that they require no machinery or equipment. They are simply-modified in that, simply by shifting the position of the body, they can be easier or more challenging to execute. And they are super-efficient in that they exercise many different muscle groups all at the same time. (Full disclosure: I used to have a hate/hate relationship with planks, but I have learned to love them for all the reasons mentioned above.)

How to do it: Place the forearms onto the mat, making sure your elbows and shoulders are in alignment. Extend one leg fully behind so that the toes are curled underneath. Extend the other leg in the same way. Drop your hips so that the body is in a straight line from head to feet. This is the traditional plank position. If you're new to planks, aim to hold the pose for ten to twenty seconds. If you're more advanced, consider trying for forty-five to sixty seconds. Remember to breathe!

Planks are a three s's exercise: straightforward, simply-modified, and super-efficient.

How to do it with baby: Your baby can be a wonderful motivator to keep you going when muscle fatigue sets in. Simply place him on his back in between your elbows. Focus on his gorgeous face and your planking will be done in no time.

How to modify it: To make a plank easier, assume the same position but hold the pose using hands on the mat instead of forearms. For a harder challenge, alternate supporting body weight between hands and forearms. Lift one forearm up and place that hand on the mat, then place the other hand on the mat. Lower the first forearm and then the second. Repeat this pattern throughout the plank hold.

Crunch & twist

Why to do it: Many of the flexercises included here are meant to provide an effective workout in a little time. As a new mother, time and energy are at a premium. So, if you choose to allocate some of them to exercise, they should be moves that really make you feel good about what you've accomplished. The crunch & twist is a challenging exercise that will target a number of core muscles, including the rectus abdominis, the obliques (a vertical set of muscles that control turning and twisting motions), and the iliopsoas (hip muscles). The crunch & twist will also benefit the quadriceps and the biceps in the arms. A set will be time well spent.

How to do it: Lie on your back with knees bent and soles of the feet on the floor. Grab a two- to three-pound dumbbell, book, or other free weight and hold it comfortably in both hands with your elbows bent and your arms extended over the head. Breathe in, and on the exhale come up to a seated position while keeping your feet firmly on the floor. The movement should be initiated from the abdominal muscles. From that seated position, twist the torso, bringing the weight to tap the floor on the left side. Then twist the torso in the opposite direction to tap the weight on the right side. Bring the weight back to center and slowly roll back down to the starting position. It may take a few tries to find the rhythm of this exercise, but then it will flow quite smoothly. Aim for ten to twelve reps.

How to do it with baby: (This exercise should only be performed with a baby who can sit up on his own.) Begin in the same starting position described above. Instead of taking a free weight, place baby on your pelvis with your hands holding her comfortably and firmly at her waist. Breathe in; exhale while coming up to a seated position. Lift baby up with both arms. Make a wide arch, bringing her to the left side, gently tapping her bottom to the floor, then back over to the right side to tap the floor. Bring her back to center and slowly recline back to the starting position.

How to modify it: To increase the difficulty level, use a heavier weight or go for fifteen reps. Ease up by skipping the weight altogether and simply tap hands on either side while performing the twisting motion.

A word on yoga and Pilates: Yoga and Pilates can be engaging, effective methods of strength training. In 2012, a market research firm cited that studios specializing in these practices are among the top ten fastest-growing industries.

Both practices lower body weight and body fat percentage, making them sound options for those interested in dropping the baby weight (Ko et al. 2013, 2122–31). An in-home Pilates exercise program decreased mental and physical fatigue in new mothers and increased activity and motivation, according to 2015 study (Ashrafina et al., 169–73). Sound good? There are numerous DVDs and classes available. Though the selection may be more limited, check out the local library to see what's on the shelves. There are

If or, perhaps more accurately, when you miss a workout, relax. Tomorrow is another day.

also numerous videos online. A word of caution: Anyone can post a video on YouTube (and I mean, anyone). If you're logging on for inspiration, make sure to choose a video with a reputable fitness instructor who knows her stuff. Use good judgment and move at an appropriate pace. Some yoga or Pilates instructors will provide in-home lessons. Forming a small group will save on the cost of the instructor and provide an opportunity to socialize before or after the class. Check out yogaalliance.org to find a local certified teacher.

If part of the motivation to work out is a mood-boost, consider keeping a mood log to examine how this tool is working for you. A mood log is quick to set up, easy to maintain, and may serve to motivate when a little something more is needed to get moving. Check out the template in the back of this book.

If or, perhaps more accurately, when you miss a workout, relax. Tomorrow is another day. This perspective can be hard to maintain in the middle of a sleep-deprived, hormonally erratic, transitional phase like becoming a mother. One of the best things you can do for yourself and your baby is to be gentle and patient with both of you. Exercise is one tool that can help in moving toward a place of greater health and well-being, but it is by far not the only one. Up next? A little *hands-on* help!

MATERNAL MASSAGE THERAPY

HANDS-ON HEALING

Touch is the mother of the senses.

—Helen Fisher, American anthropologist

Some may consider massage a luxury. Here's the reality: therapeutic touch can have healing effects on the body, and this can translate into healthier, more enjoyable living. In the weeks and months following the birth of a baby, when daily life is infused with the additional stressors of sleep deprivation, hormonal adjustments, and the learning curve of infant care, a massage can serve to enhance maternal well-being and make the day-to-day routine more manageable. Massage is a proven way to relieve and reduce stress in new mothers (Deligiannidis and

Simply put, massage makes a mom better, and that makes a better mom. Freeman 2014, 85–95). Simply put, massage makes a mom better, and that makes a better mom.

In cultures around the world postpartum massage is the norm. In India, it is not uncommon for an experienced midwife, or *Dai*, to provide a postpartum massage. Using oils such as sesame, coconut, or olive, women can enjoy the restorative benefits of a traditional massage, often followed by a warm bath. In Kuala Lumpur, the capital of Malaysia, a 2016 report confirmed that 95 percent of women who gave birth in a university hospital there received an *Urut Malayu*. This traditional postpartum wellness ritual, similar to a Swedish massage, was given within the first six or seven weeks after giving birth (Fadzil, Shamsuddin, and Puteh 2016, 505).

In Western nations, massage is among the most common of the complementary or alternative therapies used in pregnancy (Hall, Griffiths, and McKenna 2011, 818). While less frequently used in the postnatal than prenatal period, the practice offers mothers and their babies a wealth of physical and psychological benefits.

MASSAGING THE MAMA-BODY

GETTING TO KNOW MY BODY AGAIN: DARCY'S STORY

After giving birth to Malcolm, I felt like I was in someone else's body. I had a scheduled C-section after we found out that he was breech. It was my first major surgery. When I came home from the hospital, my whole body ached. Everything felt sore. Just walking around was effortful, let alone

In cultures around the world postpartum massage is the norm.

carrying Malcolm. I knew C-sections were common—women had them every day—but for me, for my body, the effects felt so overwhelming. My whole mid region throbbed. In my mind, I believed that I would heal, but I wondered and worried about how long it would take and whether I would be able to care for Malcolm in the meantime. I had pain medication from my ob-gyn; it helped a little, but I felt like I wanted something more.

When I was pregnant, my mother gave me a gift certificate for a prenatal massage. At the time, the massage therapist told me that I might consider seeing her after I gave birth as well—that it could be helpful for pain management and relaxation. I called her and she was able to come to my home for a massage treatment. What a difference! Having her healing hands on my recovering body felt so comforting. It's not like the pain went away immediately, but it did provide some relief. She taught me a few techniques I could use on myself. They were incredibly helpful throughout my healing.

As we know, pregnancy, labor, and delivery have profound and sometimes lasting effects on the body. Although many women's bodies are designed for these tasks, they are neither simple nor easy. These processes can leave scars—physical and emotional. Just as a prenatal body needs to be nurtured, so, too, does a postnatal one. Nine months of pregnancy produce dramatic physiological change. Internal organs transform, changing in size and shape. By the time of birth, the uterus, typically the size of a peach, has ballooned to the size of a watermelon! The bladder and rectum have shifted from their usual positions. The breasts have become larger (a welcome change for some, not so much for others). Your feet may have grown as much as a whole shoe size in pregnancy due to elevated growth hormones in the body. (I went from a six to a six-and-a-half size shoe in my pregnancy, and my feet have remained that half size bigger ever since.)

Then there is the actual birth experience, which varies dramatically from one woman to another. Even in the most straightforward, complication-free births, the physical task takes a toll. Muscles and ligaments that were taxed during delivery need time to heal. The area around the vagina, perineum, and rectum will be sore, and there will be residual bleeding. Complicated or traumatic labors, as well as surgical deliveries (C-sections), may result in further bodily stress. Given all of this trauma, it seems only sensible that a dose of healing touch is just what the doctor *should* order.

One of the more immediate benefits massage offers in the postpartum stage is the opportunity to decrease pain and heal more quickly. Licensed massage therapist and certified birth doula Amanda Tarver owns Women's Massage Therapy outside of Chicago. Tarver regularly sees women on the pre- and post-pregnancy spectrum. She treats clients using particular techniques to help stimulate tissue regeneration, improve elasticity, and help organs to shift back into place. Tarver points out that some women who were given an epidural during labor may be at an increased risk for damage to the soft tissue and ligaments around the hips. While the epidural dulls sensation, and therefore eases the pain of labor, it also makes it difficult to sense any strain resulting from the legs being braced or held back while baby is being born. A postpartum massage can work to ease the resulting discomfort. For her C-section clients, Tarver will take a look at the incision site and often perform therapeutic touch aimed at healing scar tissue. Specific massage maneuvers are designed to break down excess scar tissue and coax new tissue to form, thereby enhancing the appearance

One immediate benefit massage offers is the opportunity to decrease pain and heal more quickly.

and feel of the skin. In working with a postpartum client, Tarver makes use of tapping, gliding, and vibrating motions as opposed to the more traditional deep tissue techniques. These gentler approaches have the

Massage maneuvers are designed to break down excess scar tissue and coax new tissue to form.

added benefit of helping to alleviate gas and constipation, two common and often uncomfortable side-effects following birth.

Massage can also work wonders on the postnatal body when it comes to restoring posture. As pregnancy progresses and the weight of the body becomes unevenly distributed, the lower back compresses, which results in a tightening of the hip flexors (the muscles that serve to bring the knees up toward the belly). A targeted massage can help realign and retrain the muscles and ligaments to restore a more balanced stance.

Especially for first-time mothers, labor can frequently be a lengthy endeavor. Holding a position or series of positions for an extended period can cause trigger points (pain resulting from overuse of tissue) and muscle strains to develop. Postpartum massage can work to relax the muscles that may have been working overtime.

Moving past the immediate weeks after birth, moms may notice a shift in where they feel discomfort. Or worse, they may be so distracted by the newfound responsibility of motherhood that they may not notice it until it becomes almost unbearable! For mothers who are nursing, there is a tendency to hunch over while feeding baby. *Nursing neck*, as it is sometimes known, occurs when the head is folded down and the neck and shoulders are bent over for an extended period of time. A targeted massage for your neck and

A targeted massage can help realign and retrain the muscles and ligaments and restore a more balanced stance.

Postpartum massage has been proven to significantly improve sleep quality in new mothers!

shoulders can help restore comfort to the area.

Still not sold on the benefits of massage therapy? Consider this: Postpartum massage has been proven to significantly improve sleep quality in new mothers! A 2014 study published in the journal *Midwifery* reported on a group of postpartum Taiwanese women suffering from poor sleep. Participants all received the same standard postpartum care. One segment of women also received twenty-minute back massages from a certified massage therapist at the same time each evening for five consecutive days. At the end of the study, the new mothers who had received massages demonstrated significantly improved sleep over their counterparts who did not (Ko and Lee 2014, 60–64). Better sleep? That's reason enough to make postpartum massage a standard part of care for all new moms.

The American Pregnancy Association offers that postnatal massage may also contribute to maternal hormone regulation following birth. Because massage can enhance circulation, a treatment has the potential to decrease postpartum swelling, the result of a natural fluid increase during pregnancy (2015).

MASSAGING THE MAMA-MIND

Beyond the physical benefits, this healing technique also offers some proven health benefits for a mom's mental state. Numerous studies point to the feelings of relaxation many people experience during and after a massage treatment. In addition to a general sense of calm, there are particular massage applications used in the treatment of postpartum depression and postpartum post-traumatic stress disorder (PPPTSD). For some, the birth experience can be frightening, chaotic, and not what they hoped or planned for. This may be the case when a woman undergoes an emergency C-section, for instance, or experiences a life-threatening situation for herself or her baby (or both) during labor. Sometimes the feeling of being out of control or the physical sensations of the birthing process can leave one with residual anxiety or panic.

Healing touch is also a proven method of mitigating the stress that accompanies the time directly following labor. In 2014, a study was conducted on a group of women in Japan who had given birth within the past eighteen hours. Each participant had her heart rate and blood pressure recorded, as these are good indicators of the body's level of stress at a given moment. Then, one group of women was given a twenty-minute massage to the back, neck, shoulder, and hip regions. A second group of women received no massage. Measurements of heart rate and blood pressure were taken again after twenty minutes. As might be expected, a significant and favorable difference was found in the group who received the massage in contrast to the group who did not (Nakakita 2015, 87–98). The body does not lie. The mothers who received massages were more relaxed.

Massage can also be a natural and effective complement to other healing practices as well. Amanda Tarver, the owner of Women's Massage Therapy, comments that mothers who use massage treatment in combination with talk therapy tend to show remarkable improvements in recuperating during the postnatal stage (pers. comm.). (We'll explore talk therapy in greater detail in the chapter "Talk Is *Not* Cheap: The Value of Talk Therapy.")

MORE MASSAGES TO CHOOSE FROM

Massage comes in many different forms. Reflexology is one type in which the application of pressure is focused on the feet or hands. Women who received a foot massage in the first few days after delivery were found to have significantly lower levels of cortisol (the stress hormone) in their urine and reported significantly lower levels of fatigue and depressive feelings than their counterparts who did not receive the treatment (Choi and Lee 2015, 587–94). That's a pretty big pay-off for a foot rub!

In Tokyo, a group of Japanese first-time mothers were evaluated to determine the effects of aromatherapy massage. On the second day postpartum, one group of mothers each received a thirty-minute massage treatment with accompanying essential oils. In comparison to the control group, who did not receive the treatment, the mothers who accepted a massage were found to have lower feelings of anxiety and blues. The study also indicated that those mothers who received the aromatherapy massage reported feelings of greater closeness with their babies (Imura and Misao 2006, 21–27).

SELF-MASSAGE

Ideally, every new mom should be given a postpartum massage before being discharged from the hospital or birthing center, or have access to a massage therapist at home after her baby is born. Alas, that is not the case. There is, however, a wealth of massage techniques that you can practice on yourself (or that a willing partner or friend can practice on you). All of the techniques presented here offer benefits including relaxation and muscle relief. If time permits, try them all! (Wishful thinking, perhaps.) Or pick and choose the ones that target the areas in greatest need of attention on a particular day. These healing applications come by way of registered massage therapist Cassandra Hall Primeau, who works with pre- and postnatal clients at Angel Hands Integrative Centre in Vancouver, British Columbia. (The clever, or not so clever, names for the massages are my own.)

MARSUPIAL MASSAGE

Why to do it: The marsupial massage is meant to provide restoration and healing to the abdominal area where marsupials, like kangaroos, carry their young. This gentle massage can serve to help the uterus discharge any remaining tissue following birth and facilitate shrinkage of the organ back to its original size. The technique may also help with circulation to the skin around the area.

How to do it: Place both hands on the abdomen. Gently begin to move the hands in a small, circular pattern starting at the right hip and moving across to the left, then circling back to the right again. This massage may be performed during the immediate period postpartum and then daily in the weeks to follow, as it feels comfortable and therapeutic. You may perform the technique on yourself or ask your partner to do so. Note: women who had a C-section should avoid massaging the area around the incision until it is fully healed.

NURSING MOM'S MASSAGE

Why to do it: Nursing mothers will often experience periods of engorgement, when the breasts become quite full and heavy as a result of milk production. This can be rather uncomfortable (obviously). General tenderness and swelling of the breasts can be reduced through the use of targeted massage therapy.

How to do it: Place the pads of the fingers on one breast. Beginning at the nipple and moving outward, use small circular motions to knead the breast tissue. Between feedings, place a dry towel in the freezer and wrap it around the breasts in a figure eight. The cold will help bring down swelling and inflammation, and will probably feel refreshing. Frozen towel leave you (too) cold? Either keep it in the refrigerator prior to use or simply dampen it with cool water.

THE PAIN IN THE NECK MASSAGE SERIES

Why to do it: The seemingly endless hours of baby-feeding can result in some pretty poor posture. Whether nursing or bottle-feeding, there is a likelihood that you will be hunched over while snuggling with your babe. And all this hunching can wreak havoc on the muscles in your neck and shoulders, which may already be burdened as common carriers of everyday stress. Simple massage-like stretches for the neck and shoulders can help ease musculoskeletal discomfort. Do be mindful, however. There are a number of major blood vessels and nerves that run along the neck. Consider seeking out a one-on-one session with a massage therapist before trying these on your own.

How to do it: Each of the following stretches—targeting the muscles of the neck, chest, upper back, or shoulders—are most effective when held for at least thirty seconds.

- *Neck:* Slowly tilt your head to the right until your right ear is close to your right shoulder. Be sure not to raise the shoulder to the ear. Bring your right arm up and around the side of the head until your right hand is resting on your left ear. Very gently pull on the head to increase the stretch. You should feel a comfortable stretch in the back of your neck on the left side. Again, be sure that your shoulders remain comfortably in place and do not rise up. From here, gently use your right arm to bring your head from the side to the front of your body so that your nose is pointing toward your armpit. This variation enhances the initial stretch. Remember to breathe deeply through these stretches. Make sure to perform the same stretches on the other side.
- *Chest:* Clasp both hands together behind your back. Be sure not to tense up the hands when interlacing the fingers. Slowly raise your arms up and away from your

body only as high as feels comfortable. You should feel a quality stretch on either side of your upper chest. Breathe deeply while maintaining the stretch for up to thirty seconds.

- *Upper back/shoulders:* Yoga practitioners may be familiar with the following stretch known as the *eagle arms.* Place your arms straight out in front of your body. Put one elbow on top of the other elbow and then bend the arms to form a 90-degree angle. The forearms should be wrapped around each other so that the palms of the hands are touching. If this is uncomfortable, wrap your arms only to the extent that the backs of the hands touch. Slowly raise the arms up or down a few inches to where the greatest stretch may be felt in your upper back and shoulder muscles.

Again, treat yourself to some deep, cleansing breaths. Breathing is as important as the stretching itself, as it can enhance circulation and help reduce muscle tension.

There are no absolute contraindications specific to the post-partum client, instructs Cassandra; however, she advises that anyone with a serious systemic infection or fever shouldn't get a massage. Licensed practitioners should be able to make modifications or avoid direct contact or pressure to sensitive or affected areas, as in the case of a C-section scar or diastasis recti. They can also make modifications to the position in which the client is being treated in order to provide for her comfort.

INFANT MASSAGE

As with most of the other supports included in the book, massage

> Treat yourself to some deep, cleansing breaths. Breathing is as important as the stretching itself, as it can enhance circulation and help reduce muscle tension.

offers the option to include your baby in the practice. Mammals will often lick and groom their young, variations of massage, in order to enable normal bodily functioning, explains Alison Cooke, a midwife and doctoral research fellow at the University of Manchester, UK. Cooke elaborates on the long history of infant massage in Asia (where techniques are passed down from mother to daughter through the generations) and also comments that Florence Nightingale, typically credited as the mother of contemporary nursing, encouraged doctors and nurses to be trained in massage for a variety of ailments (Cooke 2015, 166–170).

Most moms who receive massage can attest to the benefits for themselves, and the research corroborates those benefits. By contrast, scientific evidence of the positive effects of massage on infants is surprisingly limited. There appears to be no hard data suggesting that properly conducted massage is harmful to babies, but plenty of anecdotal proof to support its value for both babies and moms alike.

MASSAGE AS A MEANS TO BOND: NINA'S STORY

The first weeks at home with Oscar, I kept wondering when I would feel like he was really mine. I had carried him for nine months and then given birth to him—twelve long, hard hours of labor—but somehow I just didn't feel connected. It scared me. I felt like there must be something wrong with me, like I was missing some kind of mom gene. A friend of mine invited me to an infant massage class. I went more as a favor to her, but it wound up being really great! I learned some techniques for massaging Oscar's legs and arms. He seemed to enjoy it, and so did I. It was a new way of relating to him besides holding and feeding, and there was something about the newness of it that felt refreshing. It was a nice change from the usual, daily baby care tasks. I started giving Oscar massages pretty regularly, at least once a day for the next few months. I can't be sure whether it was the massages or Oscar getting older, or me getting the hang of being a mom, but I started to feel like he was really mine.

Before beginning an infant massage, there are a few general tips to keep in mind.

RESPECTING BABY'S BODY

The masseuse, whether it be mom, dad, or caregiver, should ask baby's permission before beginning, advises Howard Steele, Professor of Psychology and Co-Director of the Center for Attachment at The New School for Social Research. This may seem strange. After all, babies cannot express their desires verbally. However, the act of asking "May I give you a massage?" demonstrates to an infant that her body is her own and that she alone should have the authority to decide if, when, and how it may be touched by another person.

As baby grows and becomes acquainted with massage, he will begin to demonstrate through body language whether he prefers to be touched at a given time. You can learn how to read and interpret the cues. Follow your baby's lead. Pay attention to how he is responding to the massage. Observing these signs can inform you about whether or not to continue the practice at a particular time. For example, does your baby's body seem more calm or active, or does he become fussy during a certain application? Remember, there are many variables that can affect a baby's response to massage—how tired he is, if he has gas, if he is hungry. If your little one does not seem to enjoy a massage the first time, it may be worth trying again on another day.

The act of asking "May I give you a massage?" demonstrates to an infant that her body is her own.

THE USE OF LUBRICANT

A second point of consideration before beginning is the use of oil. Oil can make the process of massage easier because the lubrication facilitates smoother movement over baby's limbs. If either you or your baby dislike the feel though, or if there is no suitable oil on hand, it need not be used. Those who wish to use oil should follow the recommendation of Infant Massage USA, a division of the International Association of Infant Massage. Opt for cold-pressed, unscented fruit and vegetable oils such as grapeseed, safflower, sunflower, or olive oil (n.d., par. 23). These oils are safe if ingested and are less slippery than some others. You may find it easier to dispense a small amount of oil or lotion into a bowl to have at the ready.

KEEPING BABY COMFORTABLE

Your baby may be naked or wear a diaper. Place her on her back on top of a soft blanket. Use a receiving cloth or smaller blanket over baby's chest and stomach for warmth. If you have a boy, either keep the diaper on, or else gently cover his penis—relaxation can often prompt a sprinkle! Take a moment to make sure your hands are clean and warm.

The following massages may be performed sequentially. They are described here as individual techniques for the purposes of clarity and deeper understanding. However many you decide to include, be sure to complete them fully first on one limb and then move to the opposing limb, so that both sides of the body receive the benefits. Finally, as you are performing these techniques, engaging with your baby, periodically check in with yourself. Is any tension being held in your neck, shoulders, or hands? If so, are you able to release this tension as you breathe through the movement? What impact, if any, is this activity having on your physical and emotional state? Simply notice.

INDIAN MILKING, LEG

Begin by holding one of baby's legs. Starting at the hip, place one hand on top of the other and gently squeeze and twist working downward toward the foot. The movement should be fluid and smooth, like milking a cow (hence the name), as opposed to wringing out a towel. At the foot, take a thumb and gently press into the sole while rubbing the top of the foot with the fingers. Move the thumb around the ankle joint.

SWEDISH MILKING, LEG

Similar to Indian milking, this technique uses the same type of movement but in the opposite direction. From baby's foot, gently squeeze upward back toward the hip. In her book *Infant Massage: A Handbook for Loving Parents*, Vimala McClure, founder of the International Association of Infant Massage, explains the meaning behind each of these massage techniques, both of which are used in infant massage. The tradition of Indian milking, from shoulder to wrist or in this case hip to ankle, is a symbolic act of stress and tension exiting the body. By contrast, Swedish milking reflects the idea of toning the muscles while bringing healing energy toward the heart. McClure offers that these two techniques work well together, offering a complimentary balance (2017, 147). Licensed massage therapist, Susan G. Salvo, suggests concluding the leg massage with a rolling motion and then a swift, smooth stroke. Place baby's leg between two open hands and then roll the leg between the hands, as if rolling cookie dough into a ball. Finish by placing open hands on the thigh and gently brushing the fingertips down toward the feet (Salvo 2017).

After performing the massage on both legs, check in with your baby and make some observations. How does she appear now in comparison to when the massage began? Is she calmer? More active? You might ask her if she would like to continue. In fact, you could ask yourself these same questions, too.

INDIAN MILKING, ARM

Now apply the same technique as was described above to baby's arms. Beginning at the shoulder, cup the arm in both hands and gently squeeze and twist in a downward direction toward the wrist. Massage baby's palm with your thumb while simultaneously rubbing the top of his hand with the fingertips. (Babies younger than five or six months may exhibit a palmer grasp. This is a primitive reflex in which babies will automatically close their fingers over an object placed on the palm. When newborns squeeze mom's or dad's thumb just after birth, this is the result of the palmer grasp reflex.)

SWEDISH MILKING, ARM

As with the leg, work with a gentle twisting motion, moving toward the heart. Begin at the wrist and work up closer to the shoulder, moving past the elbow. Be sure to massage the whole of the arm, front and underside. Reapply oil if necessary. Roll the arm with hands open on either side. Be sure to treat both arms.

OPEN BOOK, CHEST

Ask baby if she would like to have her chest massaged. Notice how she responds as you begin the following movement: With hands open and palms facing down, place hands side by side on the middle of baby's chest and lightly brush your hands up and over each shoulder, as if smoothing out the pages of a newspaper. Repeat this motion several times. Next, apply the *butterfly*. Begin with hands in the same starting position at the center of the chest. Instead of moving them over either shoulder simultaneously, move one hand only on a diagonal. In other words, your right hand will move up toward baby's left shoulder and back to the center of her chest. Then your left hand will move up toward baby's right shoulder and back down, as if tracing the wings of a butterfly. Repeat the butterfly several times.

WATER WHEEL/THUMBS-TO-SIDE, TUMMY

As with each previous application, ask your baby's permission to massage his belly. If baby continues to enjoy the process, and if you do as well, then it is time for some attention to the tummy. To perform the water wheel, place your hands above the belly button and perpendicular to the legs, one on top of the other. (If the belly button is not yet fully healed from birth, avoid the area.) Using the tips of the fingers, cross hand over hand lightly in a downward motion over the belly. Then, shift the hands 90 degrees so they are parallel to baby's legs. Place each thumb on his belly and move them away from each other, out toward either side of baby's body.

I-LOVE-U, FOR COLIC

The I-Love-U technique may be helpful in treating colic as it applies gentle pressure to baby's colon and bowel. Doing so can help to expel painful gas bubbles. Using the tip of the middle finger, draw a lowercase "I" (without the dot) beginning on baby's left side, just at the bottom of the rib cage. Next trace an upside down "L," beginning at the bottom of baby's rib cage on her right side, coming across and then down. Finally, make an upside down "U" motion, traveling from the baby's lower right rib cage, over the belly button, and down to the left side of the rib cage. This may be repeated several times.

KNEES TO BELLY, FOR COLIC

This is another massage that may be helpful for babies with colic. Hold baby's legs, one in each hand, and gently bend the legs at the knees so that they touch the belly. A soft wiggle when the legs are bent may enhance the movement. After a few seconds, you can either extend baby's legs back out or bring them in to the belly once or twice more if baby seems to enjoy this massage. You can also try gently rotating baby's legs in a clockwise direction beginning at her right hip, circling over to her left, and then back to her right a couple of times. This movement mirrors the direction of digestion and may help baby to release some gas, which in turn can help with colic.

WALKING FINGERTIPS, FOR GAS

This technique can help release gas bubbles in the digestive tract. Simply place your fingertips on either side of and slightly above baby's belly button. Gently tap or "walk" the fingers around the area. This may be followed by a few more water wheel movements. (See above.)

BACK & FORTH, BACK

Lift baby up and place her face down across your thighs, as if she were preparing for some tummy-time. With hands placed palms down flat on baby's back, slowly move each hand forward and back in opposite directions. After a moment, take baby's feet in your right hand. With the left hand, begin at baby's neck and glide down the length of baby's body. If she permits, gently begin the motion again starting at the back of her head.

> At this moment in life, the power of touch can be harnessed to provide healing and restoration.

Applying massage on such a little being can feel a bit nerve-wracking. You may be wondering if you are applying sufficient pressure, for example. Taking an infant massage class, offered in some hospitals, or watching an infant massage video will be a great help. For a wonderful video of Susan Salvo demonstrating infant massage, check the link in the Resources section. Brandi Jordan, MSW, a board-certified lactation consultant and newborn care specialist, offers some helpful advice and lovely demos as well. A link to her video can also be found in the Resources section. With a little bit of practice, you will grow comfortable, and you and your baby may find you both enjoy the experience greatly.

The English poet John Keats wrote that "touch has a memory." Indeed. The impact of touch, good or bad, leaves an indelible impression on the body whether one is fully conscious of it or not. At this moment in life, the power of touch can be harnessed to provide healing and restoration. Use it thoughtfully now to create an archive of lasting and comforting memories for both you and your child.

In the same way touch leaves a memory on the body, the tool detailed in the following chapter can "up the ante," enabling positive and lasting change on both the body and the mind. If you're ready to reduce your maternal stress and enhance your happiness, you're ready to meditate.

MEDITATION

OM AWAY THE BABY BLUES AND SOME OTHER THINGS, TOO

You can't stop the waves, but you can learn to surf.
—Jon Kabat-Zinn, American scientist,
writer, and meditation teacher

Meditation has become something of an umbrella term, a word referring to any one of a number of different exercises, often intended to enable one's spiritual and overall well-being. Some form of meditation exists in *every* major world religion, writes clinical psychologist and marriage counselor Robert Puff (2013). He asserts that meditation can be of great benefit to everyone, regardless of the faith with which she identifies or if she identifies with any faith (2013).

> Meditation, then, is an excellent tool to employ when time and energy are at a premium. By its very nature, it is a practice that requires no *doing*, but rather simply *being*.

As a new mother, meditation can hold tremendous power as an instrument for moving through the challenges of daily life. This is due at least in part to the relative ease with which meditation can be practiced. The exercises included later in the chapter can all be done in any place at any time. This means that a mother might engage in a few moments of meditative practice while she is nursing or pumping, for example, or while her baby is in the swing or Pack 'n' Play or even in a carrier attached to her body. Meditation, then, is an excellent device to employ when time and energy are at a premium. By its very nature, it is a practice that requires no *doing*, but rather simply *being*.

Not unlike massage, there are many different kinds of meditation that may be practiced in many different ways. There are meditations that derive from the Buddhist tradition, such as Zen and Vipassana. There are those meditations steeped in Hindu philosophy, such as mantra (Om) meditation and Transcendental Meditation (TM). There are also a wide variety of yoga practices which incorporate meditation. Some of these include Kundalini Yoga and Kriya. At some point, it may be worth exploring the various kinds of meditation that exist, as one size does not fit all. But that time is probably not now. Now is the time for a simple, effective tool to help make the day-to-day job as a mom more manageable. So, the focus here will be on one specific form of meditative practice: mindfulness, because this one has been scientifically proven to reduce some of the most common struggles that arise postpartum.

WHY MEDITATE NOW? HOW MEDITATION HELPS NEW MOMS

Meditation may be the ticket to greater self-love and lower self-criticism. (Doesn't that sound delightful!) Mindfulness-Based Stress Reduction (MBSR) is a particular form of meditation that incorporates elements of mindfulness (for more on mindfulness, see the chapter "Feed Me! Healing Meals for Mamas") and yoga. After receiving instruction and taking part in this meditation exercise, a group of new moms in Spain reported significantly higher feelings of self-compassion and maternal self-efficacy, a belief in one's own ability to mother, as well as lower stress and anxiety levels than they had before (Blasco, Viguer, and Rodrigo 2013, 227). Worth noting is the fact that each individual meditation session was relatively short—ten minutes—and that they were all conducted with babies present.

A second study introduced an eight-week mindfulness-based meditation program for mothers during the last half of pregnancy and into the postpartum period. Though the sample size was small, thirty-one moms, the results indicate that those who meditated showed significantly reduced anxiety and negative emotion than the control group (Vieten and Astin 2008, 67).

For women with a history of depression prior to or during pregnancy, mindfulness-based meditation may be an especially important tool in preserving good mental health in the perinatal period. A group of pregnant women with previous histories of depression were enrolled in a Mindfulness-Based Cognitive Therapy (MBCT) program. Cognitive therapy is a type of talk therapy that focuses on the ways thoughts influence feelings.

Therefore, MBCT combines aspects of mindfulness-based meditation and cognitive therapy to effectively reduce the likelihood of depression reoccurring. The women in the program who received MBCT had significantly lower rates of depression recurrence or depressive symptoms postpartum than those who were receiving other types of mental health treatment or no treatment at all (Dimidjian et al. 2016, 140–41).

MANAGING MAJOR TRANSITIONS: MELISSA'S STORY

I had a difficult time my freshman year of college. I was very close to my parents growing up and felt extremely homesick when I moved into the dorm. The school was so big, it seemed impossible to really get to know anybody. When I came home for the Thanksgiving holiday, I told my parents how lonely I was and that I didn't feel like going back to school. We agreed that I would speak with a counselor at the campus health clinic and that if I was still feeling badly by the end of the fall term, I could take the spring semester off and think about transferring. I was lucky in that I found a really great therapist with whom I connected. She really helped support me through the transition to college-life, teaching me some meditative techniques that I could use when I was feeling anxious and overwhelmed. She helped me learn ways to feel more relaxed and at ease. Slowly, I started to find my people and settle in to college life.

When I got pregnant with my daughter, I remember starting to feel very nervous about the changes ahead. I wanted to be a mom, but as my due date approached, I just became more and more anxious. I was really scared that I would slip into another depression, and I couldn't imagine how I would take care of my baby in that state. I revisited the practices I used in college and started going to a mindfulness-meditation class at a local yoga studio. After each class, I could feel my whole body just sort of exhale. I keep up a daily meditation practice to this day. Sometimes I only get five or ten minutes in, but it makes a big difference.

Adopting a meditative practice can not only make the work of mothering less stressful, as it did for Melissa, but it can also (along with some other techniques we will explore in the chapter "And Baby Makes Three: How Bringing Baby Home Can Bring a Couple Closer Together") strengthen the ability of you and your partner to work together as co-parents.

A 2015 study explored the effects of couples who participated in a mindfulness-based relationship education program. The couples, all of whom were expecting a first child, reported that taking part in the program "deepened connections with their partners and led them to be more confident about becoming parents" (Gambrel and Piercy, 25). Incidentally, male partners reported feeling a greater identification with fatherhood after taking part in the mindfulness program.

MEDITATION FOR NEW PARENTS: TORI'S STORY

Shawn and I were so happy when we found out I was pregnant. After two unsuccessful rounds of IVF, the third one was the lucky charm. Looking back now, I think that because we had such a hard time trying to conceive, all of our focus was on getting pregnant and we didn't think too much about what might happen after that. As the weeks progressed, we both felt a bit anxious—first about being able to maintain the pregnancy and then about actually having a baby! One of our fertility doctors told us about a support group for couples taking place at the hospital. She said that it might be a good way to help manage the transition to becoming parents and allevi-ate some of the anxiety. We had our doubts—we had never been in any sort of a support group before, but we trusted our doctor, so we gave it a try. The first few weeks of the program we learned about some mindfulness-meditation techniques to help lower stress and feel more relaxed and calm. We learned about ways of prac-ticing kindness and patience. In the last few weeks, we tried out some techniques to better understand how our partner may be feel-ing and how to be more sensitive in talking about issues where we disagree. I thought it was pretty interesting, but the biggest surprise was Shawn. He loved it! We are now expecting our second child and Shawn will often use a technique that we learned in the group when we are feeling overwhelmed or need to reconnect. Learning those mindfulness meditation skills was one of the best things we did together as parents.

Carla Naumburg, a writer, clinical social worker, and mother, has written a number of books on the subjects of meditation and moth-erhood and writes the *Mindful Parenting* blog for PsychCentral .com. Based on the work of MBSR pioneers Jon Kabat-Zinn and Amy Saltzman, Naumburg offers a simple and beautiful definition of mindfulness. She defines it as the act of "setting an intention to pay attention in the present moment, with kindness and curi-osity, so we can then choose our next action or behavior" (2015, par. 10). There is quite a lot of meaning packed into those words. Naumburg breaks the definition down into more digestible bites. The first part, "setting an intention," is really about making a choice. As a mom, you make millions of choices every day. You choose the onesies to dress your baby in, what to make for lunch, when to eat it, whether or not to go out for a walk or try and get some rest, and on and on and on. In the case of mindful meditation, an intention is the *conscious* choice to focus on a chosen thing—one thing. That may be focusing on one's breathing or the act of washing a bottle, but the point is to make a purposeful decision to draw attention to that act and that act only. (My latest attempt at setting an intention is to focus on the bowl of cereal I'm about to eat for breakfast. I can't prove it, but when I am able to do so, I think it tastes just a bit better.)

In the second part of her definition, Naumburg refers to "pay[ing] attention." Following the act of setting an intention, the next step is actually doing it! Really paying attention to something can be both simple and complex. A six-month-old, for example, may be mesmerized by a game of peekaboo. She may engage with complete dedication, but only until something else catches her attention. In mindful meditation, paying attention involves noticing where your focus is at a given moment. Is it on the intended thing, the act of bottle-washing or of breathing? Or has it shifted to something else? Paying attention means choosing to bring *attention* back to the *intention*. Just as a baby's focus will shift to something of greater interest, so, too, will her mother's. In mindfulness, paying attention refers to the act of noticing and, often, redirecting focus. Particularly in the early stages of mindful meditation practice, redirecting focus is usually the biggest challenge. In a culture filled with perpetual distraction, training the brain to adopt a singular concentration is no easy feat. The good news is that, as with all other skills, practice can make, if not perfect, much, much better.

An especially important aspect of mindful meditation refers to what Naumburg defines as "kindness and curiosity." To a new mother, these

> Training the brain to adopt a singular concentration is no easy feat. The good news is that, as with all other skills, practice can make, if not perfect, much, much better.

Practicing kindness toward yourself is not something women are often taught to do, but it should be. are concepts worthy of spending some time on. So often, mothers are judged, reprimanded, or devalued. So often, maternal self-talk revolves around a refrain of could-haves and should-haves. Practicing kindness toward yourself is not something women are often taught to do, but it should be. Imagine if, instead of immediately defaulting to self-criticism about a particular thought or action, you approached it with curiosity? What if, rather than saying, "I should not have done that," you began with "*Why* did I do that?" Curiosity in mindful meditation creates space, space to allow a mother to get to better know and understand her maternal self. In so doing, she can begin to figure out how she operates as a mom—which aspects of mothering bring great pleasure and which bring great challenge, which skills bring feelings of competence and which may benefit from more time and experience.

Beginning to observe yourself with kindness and curiosity informs the final part of Naumburg's explanation of mindfulness. The notion of mindfully "choosing action or behavior" is about learning to place attention on what is happening in the present moment. This may seem simple, but most people find it challenging to focus exclusively on one activity, especially in today's world. The good news is that the brain can be trained, or taught, to begin to shift attention to the here and now and let past or future concerns drift away. And, as was mentioned at the start of the chapter, learning to do so can bring great rewards for the maternal mind and body, including stress reduction, enhanced sleep, and a healthier relationship between co-parents.

MINDFULNESS MEDITATIONS FOR MOMS

Though there are a wide variety of meditative practices, the ones presented here are rooted in mindfulness philosophy for a number of reasons: they are simple to learn (though this should not be confused with being easy to practice), they have been proven effective in reducing some of the common stressors associated with postpartum life, and they may be performed nearly anytime, anywhere, with or without your baby. In exploring them remember two of the main tenets of mindful meditation: kindness and curiosity.

A MINDFUL ATTITUDE

Why to do it: As a new mom, time takes on a different quality. In one way, the days may feel endless: an ongoing monotony of feeding, changing, and napping. In another way, there may not seem to be enough time—time to sit for a leisurely dinner, time to exercise, time for those activities you enjoyed before baby came. This exercise may be useful at any point, but perhaps especially so on those days when you are craving some me-time (or mom-time) and are finding it hard to come by. A mindful attitude offers an opportunity to begin to hone the skills of mindful meditation and ideally reap the benefits without having to commit a big chunk of the day.

How to do it: Choose a common activity, one that may be performed on a regular basis such as brushing your teeth or washing the dishes. (If you are using a breast pump, consider trying this exercise while washing those seemingly infinite parts.) Make a conscious decision to place your focus exclusively on the exercise. While brushing your teeth, for example, pay attention to the taste of the toothpaste or the feel of the bristles on your pearly whites or the handle in your hand. For those few minutes, that is all that is happening. As other thoughts filter into your mind, acknowledge their presence and then redirect your attention to the task at hand: teeth-brushing, dish-washing, or other chosen activity.

SIT DOWN AND BREATHE

Why to do it: Focusing on your breath is a common entry point to many different kinds of meditative practice. Because everyone breathes (hopefully!) the breath offers an accessible portal by which you can enter meditation. More so, developing an awareness of breath can provide the opportunity to help you notice, and then regulate, moments of heightened anxiety or tension. For this exercise, adapted from Dr. Naumburg, the main purpose is to try and quiet down the mind in order to be more present.

How to do it: Sit in a comfortable chair or on a cushion on the floor. Lying down is also an option. (Be aware, lying down may well result in a nap rather than a meditation. This, of course, will offer a different set of benefits.) If you have your baby with you, you can hold her in your arms or in a carrier. This can be a soothing exercise as baby is settling into a nap after nursing perhaps. Begin with several deep breaths. Then simply allow the body to take the lead with the breath, settling into its own rhythm. Make a choice to place attention on your breath, either noticing the air passing in and out of the nose, or inflating and deflating the belly. (If the abdominal region is sore following a C-section, you may breathe in to the discomfort and notice if it provides relief, or instead choose to shift your attention away from the area.) In order to help keep focus on the breath, try counting breaths up to ten and then begin the count again. Or, quietly say "in" and "out" in sync with the motion of the breath. The mind will wander away. This is a natural part of the process, as this is exactly what the mind is used to doing. In a gentle way, redirect your attention back to the flow of air. Try setting a timer for twenty minutes. Or ten. Or five. Or however long feels manageable, especially in the beginning. Most importantly, do not judge how well or poorly the meditation was performed. In this case, the process is more important than the result (Naumburg 2015).

MINDFUL AWARENESS OF BREATHING

Why to do it: Cassandra Vieten has researched and written extensively on the subjects of motherhood and mindfulness-based meditation. Her book *Mindful Motherhood* includes a variety of mindfulness-based exercises for new and expectant moms. Dr. Vieten offers wonderful meditations, including the following, which may also be accessed for free as a guided audio recording (see link in Resources). This exercise is a reminder that breathing is always happening in the now and that learning to place focus on the breath is a way of bringing the whole of oneself into the present, a concept which is at the very heart of mindful meditation practice. Breathing happens automatically without you needing to *do* anything. As a new mother, so rare are those instances of not needing to be doing something.

Dr. Vietan offers that this exercise can enable the process of learning to allow experiences to simply happen with awareness, without needing to work at them in

> Breathing happens automatically without you needing to *do* anything. As a new mother, so rare are those instances of not needing to be doing something.

the way in which we may be familiar. She suggests that developing a mindful awareness of breathing may be especially challenging (and, one might infer, especially useful) for those moms who are typically do-ers. Indeed, the practice necessitates a slowing down and this can feel initially uncomfortable for many people (like myself) who are inclined to go-go-go. "[It is] only from the place of allowing things to be as they are," says Vieten, "[of] meeting them fully, that [you] can make intentional choices about how to respond to each situation" (2011). When you try this exercise, consider what it might be like to simply be an impartial observer, as opposed to the participant. Perhaps this will help.

How to do it: Take a moment to bring awareness to the spine, making any needed adjustments so that it is straight but not stiff. As the spine lifts to straighten, the rib cage should expand to allow the belly to rise and fall freely. Notice that the shoulders are not tensed up and the chin and jaw are relaxed. If it feels comfortable, gently turn the corners of the mouth slightly upward in a subtle smile. Breathe through the nose. Notice where in the body you feel your breath most strongly—in your belly, at your nostrils, or in your chest, for example—and shift your attention to that area. Dr. Vieten uses a beautiful metaphor for placing attention: it is not a sharp turn of focus, but rather a "butterfly landing."

If your baby is in your lap or attached to your chest, you may notice his breathing as well as your own. Perhaps your breathing is synchronized. Perhaps not. Simply notice. Thoughts will flutter in. Observe them without judgment, then let them slip away while bringing focus gently back to the flow of air. Briefly scan your posture. Notice if your spine could benefit from a little lift, or if your shoulders might enjoy a downward release. Follow the circle of the breath from the inhalation through to the exhalation and again, from the inhalation to the exhalation. Notice and acknowledge when your mind wanders off. Gently return your attention back to the flow of the breath circle. If your feel discomfort in your body, you have a choice: you can either breathe in to that discomfort or shift your position.

There is one task here, awareness. Awareness of both your own breath and your child's. There is no need to *do* or to *try*. Notice any feelings. Fatigue. Relaxation. Agitation. Allow them to be present without pressure to do anything about them. As your breathing flows without resistance, so too should these feelings pass through, without interference or judgment. Welcome the breath to deepen still and fill the whole body, breathing into the arms and legs. Bring the full body awareness to your baby as well, whether he is physically with you or not. Give respect to yourself, honoring the time you have dedicated to the practice. Take a nice stretch and a few more deep breaths. Open your eyes (Vieten 2011).

Like all the tools in this book, mindful meditation is one that continues to be beneficial long after your baby grows up. At any place, at any time, this is a vehicle that may be used to help bring you back to the here and now, back to yourself. This is also a practice that may be explored with others. Many opportunities exist to practice meditation together, from local classes (often yoga studios will offer meditation workshops) to week- or sometimes month-long retreats. Attending a class with others provides a chance to develop meditative practice and experience the powerful energy of engaging in this discipline with others. While this may not be possible at the present time, it may be an option for later. Check the Resources section for places that offer retreats.

> Like all the tools in this book, mindful meditation is one that continues to be beneficial long after your baby grows up. At any place, at any time, this is a vehicle that may be used to help bring you back to the here and now, back to yourself.

As we have learned, meditation is also a practice that couples may engage in together, and it can be a valuable resource when stress is high and patience is in short supply. In fact, there are many ways that couples can learn to minimize the challenges of early parenting or, at least, manage them more effectively. This time in a relationship can be an entrée into a more meaningful connection. Bringing home a baby can actually bring a couple closer together.

AND BABY MAKES THREE

HOW BRINGING BABY HOME CAN BRING A COUPLE CLOSER TOGETHER

Being married is like having somebody permanently
in your corner. It feels limitless, not limited.

—Gloria Steinem, American writer and feminist organizer

T hat familiar expression "two's company, three's a crowd" may never be more fitting than after a couple brings home a baby. For all the joys parenting bestows, the introduction of this new family member can also leave a lot less space for couple-dom. Or does it? Armed with a little knowledge and a few skills, this particular time in a relationship can present a rich opportunity to create a stronger, more connected partnership. Building a more solid bond now will not only benefit you as an individual, but will benefit your baby, as well, through the establishment of an environment that feels safe and secure.

Tending to a baby is a full-time job. This can make reserving time to tend to your mother-self a challenge, and finding time to tend to a partner nearly impossible. Surprisingly though, a little bit of attention can go a long way toward fortifying a relationship. Although patience and sympathy reserves may be in short supply, small, well-timed gestures can diffuse some of the stress both parents experience. Instead of feeling angry or resentful toward a partner, the potential exists to feel deeply supported and cared for. This potential can have a big payoff when it comes to keeping the *happy* in the marriage.

CAN'T WE ALL JUST GET ALONG: FAIR-FIGHTING

I'M THE MOM!: YUKO'S STORY

Early in our courtship, I remember thinking that Jake would be an incredible father. We talked about having kids when things got serious. Soon after we were married, we were thrilled to find out I was pregnant. Jake was very involved after Alexander was born. He was up in the middle of the night to change diapers and dress him. He took him out for walks on weekends. He also had very specific ideas about how things should be done. We disagreed on all sorts of matters, from which stroller to buy to where to put the bassinet. So many items had to be negotiated and, more often than not, a simple conversation about what to pack in the diaper bag would erupt into a huge fight about—I can't even remember what! I love Jake, and I am lucky he is such a caring father. Once in a while though, I fantasize about making decisions on my own, without feeling obligated to consult him. I know Jake is Alex's parent, too, and his feelings are valid, but sometimes I just want to yell at him and say, "I'm his mother! I know better!" Lately, it seems like we fight more and more. I miss how easy it used to be between us.

One of the most common complaints new parents confess about their relationship post-baby is an increase in poor communication. Simply put, when a baby comes along, quite often so too does the bickering. Between the lack of sleep and the stress of the baby-care learning curve, maintaining a sense of calm and cool when tempers flare can be an exercise in futility.

Yuko and Jake are like so many new parents who find that the dynamic of their relationship shifts abruptly after bringing home a baby. Though it may be hard to admit, many moms and dads report a decline in marital satisfaction after a child is born. In her illuminating best-seller *All Joy and No Fun*, author Jennifer Senior explores a number of large-scale studies that point to the inverse relationship between parenting and happiness in coupledom. The proof is in the research. When a baby comes along there is often a real dip in marital contentedness—at least for a while (2014, 3–6).

Certainly, it is unrealistic to believe that fighting can (or even should) be completely eliminated, but it can be reduced. As a mom, feeling buoyed by a co-parent can work wonders for a sense of overall well-being, which points to the importance of learning to communicate more thoughtfully and effectively. Learning to

One of the most common complaints new parents confess about their relationship post-baby is an increase in poor communication. Simply put, when a baby comes along, quite often so too does the bickering.

express yourselves in this manner will have positive effects well into the future.

THE FAIR-FIGHT TECHNIQUE

Why to do it: Fighting is an essential and healthy part of relationships, particularly long-term ones. The key is knowing how to fight fairly and productively. While it may be difficult to remember how to argue effectively in the heat of the moment, these are skills that can be learned, practiced, and improved upon. We may be able to forgive each other for the things we say in anger, but having enough awareness and control to stop ourselves from saying them in the first place serves us better in the long run.

How to do it: Learning to quarrel fairly, or perhaps more accurately, how to fight lovingly, requires practice, but the rewards are well worth it. Here are a series of exercises (that may be used separately or together) to test out the next time a clash is brewing.

Come back to the body

When you are upset, your body changes physiologically. While individual responses vary from one person to another, some of the most common symptoms include an increase in muscle tension, clenching of the hands and jaw, and feeling hot. Your breathing may quicken. Learn to recognize what is happening in your own body when anger bubbles up. Slow down your respiration by taking a deep breath in through your nose and exhaling out through the mouth. Notice any muscle tension and try to release it through flexing or moving your muscles (i.e., opening and closing your hands or massaging your jaw bone). Since the body and mind are connected, calming your body's response can help you to calm your emotional response as well, and this can enable you to more clearly express yourself.

Take a time-out

When we speak of motherhood, the phrase *time-out* is usually associated with disciplining a toddler. The problem with trying to communicate when tempers rise is that it becomes almost impossible to speak or listen successfully. When it comes to arguing, a time-out can be an excellent tool for short-circuiting a screaming match that feels out of control or, better yet, stopping it before it reaches critical mass. Both partners reserve the right to call a time-out at any point in the conversation. When one or the other does so, each person should go to a different space—the bedroom, kitchen, living room. A walk around the block is also an option. Take ten or fifteen minutes apart. Use the separation to calm your body (see above), take a few sips of water, and cool off. The conflict can always be revisited at a later time after the dust has settled a bit.

Create a safe space

Even the strongest partnerships can be tested by the stress of a new baby. If either of you feels like things are off-kilter in the relationship, consider the gift of couples' counseling. Many people wonder why they need therapy, especially if they have supportive friends and family members. At times of stress, like early parenthood, sometimes a different kind of help is required. A trained, experienced couples' therapist can offer something that even the closest friends and family members cannot: a reliable, safe, impartial, and non-judgmental space for partners to work through their conflicts. In spite of their best intentions, loved ones often harbor strong opinions and biases of which they may not always be aware. Though they may mean well, their judgments may be clouded. Having a regular place to go to work through domestic issues can serve to create a much happier, healthier place to come home to.

A trained, experienced couples' therapist can offer something that even the closest friends and family members cannot: a reliable, safe, impartial, and non-judgmental space for partners to work through their conflicts.

If maternal happiness is not incentive enough to seek support, consider your baby. Babies are incredibly sentient beings. Even if parents are not screaming at the top of their lungs in front of a little one (and if they are, they should consider what affect that might be having on him), babies can and do pick up on others' feelings. This does not mean that mom has to be a ball of sunshine around her baby every second of every day. That is just not reality. What it does mean is this: If you, or your partner, is screaming, crying, sulking, frowning, or ignoring the other on a regular basis, this may be creating a chaotic, scary, and insecure home for your little one. The environment to which people are exposed in early childhood affects the rest of their lives. Adults can usually make a choice to establish more pleasant surroundings for themselves. Babies get what they get, and they are stuck with it unless their parents make a change. Every mom deserves to be in a home that feels safe and loving, and so does every baby.* If a parenting partnership is not feeling how it should, the time to change it is now.

---

* A note on violence: No person should feel compelled to be in a home where personal safety is at risk. If a family member is abusive, there is help available through the National Domestic Violence Hotline: 1-800-799-SAFE (7233). For more information, visit the National Coalition Against Domestic Violence website at www.ncadv.org.

GETTING BACK BETWEEN THE SHEETS: POSTPARTUM SEX AND ROMANCE

NO INTEREST (AT THE MOMENT): CATHERINE'S STORY

Joe and I enjoyed a great sex life. We had some issues, like all couples I guess, but the bedroom was never one of them. We satisfied each other in bed and usually wanted it when the other person did, even throughout my pregnancy. When Hope was born, we were both so excited, but I felt a pretty abrupt shift in my libido. Joe said I was the "sexiest Mama he'd ever seen," but I had never felt less attractive in my life. I felt fat, tired, and kind of leaky, not to mention the fact that every ounce of energy I had was focused on Hope. "Maybe things will get better after my six-week follow-up," I thought. But when I reached that six-week mark, even though my ob-gyn said I could have sex whenever I was ready, I just had zero interest. Every time Joe came close to me I shooed him away. And then I began to worry. I mean, I knew he had needs too. How much of this could he put up with? I had read about a couple's sex life going down-hill after a baby comes along, but I never would have believed it would happen to me and Joe.

Many couples experience a change in their sexual relationship after a baby joins the family. Apart from the sleep deprivation, which is enough to make most people choose rest over sex, babies have a way of coming between their parents, literally. Making space for physical intimacy can be especially challenging when, for example, your baby is co-sleeping with you. Even if he is not in your bed but is in your room, the idea of sex may feel uncomfortable.

Happily, there are a number of ways to keep the romance alive during the postpartum period and beyond. Here are some tools to turn up the heat when a once fiery romance feels like it's dwindling.

THE ROMANCE, REINVENTED (RR) TECHNIQUE

Why to do it: There will be a period of time, especially in the first weeks postpartum, when traditional sex is contraindicated. The vagina needs time to heal from labor and delivery. For moms who delivered via C-section, the abdominal region will be sore and the incision site needs to remain clean and undisturbed. This can be an ideal opportunity to be creative in the approach to showing affection for one other. Another way to think about RR, a series of exercises, is as a sort of prolonged foreplay serving as an exciting build-up to the main event which may take place later on.

How to do it: RR is comprised of several different activities which may be used in any combination.

Turn on the flirt

Each couple has a unique history of dating rituals, patterns of activity once used to woo one another. This is a perfect time to revisit some of those tried and tested techniques and perhaps employ some new ones.

Remember dating? Each couple has a unique history of dating rituals, patterns of activity once used to woo one another. This is a perfect time to revisit some of those tried and tested techniques and perhaps employ some new ones. It worked once before and it can work again. The following acts can serve up some *sexy* in a super-short time:

Send a text message with your honeymoon destination and the caption "Remember what we did here?"

Email a love poem or sonnet (borrow one from Shakespeare or craft an original for bonus points!).

Leave a sticky (love) note on a brown bag lunch or brief case.

Linger a little longer on a good-bye kiss.

Get in the abstain game

Sometimes the biggest turn-on is being forced to turn it off, at least for a little while. In certain yoga and religious practices, sexual abstinence is believed to enable and enhance spiritual enlightenment. Besides, there are a whole lot of ways to be physically intimate short of intercourse. Consider the baseball metaphor for foreplay: first base (kissing), second base (fondling), etc. Take batting practice and hit a few singles and doubles for a while. Save a home run for later in the season.

Commit to date night or date day

Realistically, getting a night out away from a newborn is not always possible. If securing Grandpa, Aunt Sue, or a reliable sitter is feasible, do it! If it is not, don't fret. A date is still very doable, it may simply require some creativity and flexibility.

When your baby is sleeping, grab the monitor and go into the bedroom. If she sleeps in your bedroom, go into the den or other comfortable space. Power down electronics. Focus on one another. A great exercise to get you going is a series of questions by the psychologist Arthur Aron that can be found online and printed out. (See the link in the Resources section). Don't worry

Date "nights" need
not take place
at night. Think
afternoon delight!

about answering all thirty-six questions. Just enjoy the process of falling
in love again.

Date "nights" need not take place
at night. Think afternoon delight! It
may be easier to secure childcare during the day. Meet at the office
for a lite lunch together (and maybe dessert?). Consider going out
for weekend brunch or an early-bird special at a favorite neigh-
borhood hot spot.

WHEN THE TIME COMES

When you do feel ready for the main event, here are a few tips to
ease the re-entry shock:

- *Go slow.* This may seem obvious, but it's worth a gentle
  reminder to your partner to be mindful about the pace
  and to proceed with care.
- *Be realistic in your expectations.* This time around is
  unlikely to be the best sex of your life. Focus on expand-
  ing intimacy. Connect with your partner through
  eye contact, kissing, and hugging around and during
  intercourse.
- *If at first you don't succeed . . .* You may find that the first
  attempt after birth is too uncomfortable to be enjoyable.
  Baby steps. Eliminate any pressure to reach full penetra-
  tion or to climax. Focus on creating sensations that do
  feel good. You may even discover some new favorites!

BRINGING UP BABY: HOW TO SHARE IN THE CARE

ALL WORK, ALL THE TIME: MELINDA'S STORY

Paul took so much pride when he finished Jordan's crib the day before I went into labor! He was at every prenatal checkup appointment with me and was so helpful getting the nursery in order. After we brought Jordan home, though, there was so much more to do, and we both had less energy to do it. When Paul went back to work two weeks later, he was even less available. He would come home exhausted at the end of the day, and all I would want to do was hand Jordan over to him because I was exhausted myself. We were two grown-ups and one baby. A two-to-one ratio seemed like it should be enough, but we always felt like there was more to do than we could do ourselves. I knew it would be a lot of work, and I was expecting to be tired, but I had no idea how much until I was right in the middle of it—drowning.

Early motherhood (and fatherhood, too) can be made easier through prioritization. Some of this will happen automatically; there will no longer be time or energy to debate which cereal to have for breakfast. Other choices can be made more strategically. A little mental planning-ahead can save a lot of time later on and can spare you and your partner some unnecessary stress. When it's possible, delegating baby care beyond the both of you will

> A little mental planning-ahead can save a lot of time later on and can spare you and your partner a lot of unnecessary stress.

also free both people to spend a bit more time together as a couple. Quality time together has the power to strengthen the bonds of both parenthood and your relationship. So how can you begin prioritizing? Of course caring for your little one is at the top of the list, but the following guide can help you in deciding where to draw the line beyond that and how to stick to it.

POSTPARTUM PRIORITIZATION TECHNIQUE (PPT)

Why to do it: For most new moms there is not much choice. Unless endless help is available and affordable (my wish for every mom), prioritization is a must. Even if it is available, nursing moms are bound to be up at all hours, and the sleep disruption will make it harder to function during the day.

How to do it: Here are a group of straightforward, easy-to-use tips for figuring out what is most important to do (or *not* do) beyond baby care.

Pick and choose chores

If you were a Type A personality before baby, you may have been used to getting all the laundry, dishes, and grocery shopping done in one shot. The postpartum period can wreak havoc on a Type A personality. Determine which chore is most important and commit to that one and that one *only*. Pick one a day and rotate through them. At the end of the week, you will have some unwashed laundry, some dishes still in the sink, and a partially stocked fridge, but you will also be a little more rested and relaxed, and that's worth a whole lot more right now.

*Forgo Facebook (and Snapchat and Instagram
and Twitter and . . .)*

When your babe is sleeping peacefully and there are a few minutes
to spare, consider the best use of this sacred quiet time. In a culture
that is perpetually plugged-in, people often find themselves glued
to the screen without even being fully conscious of it. Consider
using one of the tools in this book, enjoy a cup a tea while flipping
through a favorite magazine, reading a newspaper (remember
those?), or just collapsing on the couch for a few moments. Your
over-stimulated mind and body will appreciate the chance to rest.

Delegate, delegate, delegate

The phrase "it takes a village" may be cliché, but the fact remains:
baby-raising requires all hands on deck, or at least as many reliable ones as are available. If your family and friends offer to help,
accept it. If they don't, then ask them for it. Be specific about what
you need. If your sister is willing to go grocery shopping, cook,
clean, or run a few errands, then sign her up. Certainly if anyone
in the clan is particularly good with babies, consider letting him
take a turn with childcare so you can have a break. If your family is
far away or unreliable, consider calling in a professional if budget
allows. Not sure who to call? Here's a quick breakdown of who is
trained to help with what:

- *The Lactation Consultant:* For some, nursing is a fairly
  seamless process that results in a well-fed baby and a
  blissful mother. For many of us, it doesn't work that
  way. Some moms who choose to breastfeed encounter
  an enormously challenging, even painful, experience. An

Internationally Board-Certified Lactation Consultant (IBCLC) is trained in educating mothers and babies on breastfeeding techniques and problem-solving. Lactation consultants will usually come to the home and offer private sessions on how to breastfeed effectively. To find one in the community, see the Resources section in the back of the book.

Keep in mind that even the most gifted lactation consultant may not be able to alleviate the difficulty for every woman. If you are struggling to breastfeed, consider the value in preserving your overall health and well-being, as well as the importance of these in maintaining solid relationships with your partner and your child. Nursing is only one way among others to bond with your baby and to provide sound nutrition.

- *The Baby Nurse:* Baby nurses are non-medical personnel who have professional experience in caring for newborns. They will come to the home and often provide either twenty-four-hour assistance or twelve-hour (night shift) coverage for a newborn. Baby nurses may live in or out depending on the needs of the family. For some couples, the baby nurse can be a lifesaver (or at least a marriage saver) during those first few weeks. As with all outside help, there are pros and cons to consider when thinking about hiring a baby nurse. Particularly for parents having a first child or those couples who may have limited-to-no experience with newborns, a baby nurse can provide concrete help, some emotional reassurance, and a temporary respite from baby care when it is most needed.

  On the flip side, not everyone is comfortable having a stranger come in and perhaps live in their homes for a concentrated period of time, particularly those living in an apartment or small space. If a baby nurse sounds like an appealing option, make sure to hire one through a reputable agency that vets its employees thoroughly. Ask a lot of questions and get references.

- *The Postpartum Doula:* Similar to a birth doula who provides support during labor and delivery, a postpartum doula offers help in the days and weeks after bringing baby home. While there are some similarities to a baby nurse, the focus of the postpartum doula is to provide assistance to the mother, father, and older siblings (if there are any) through the transition. She might offer some guidance around breastfeeding, for example, but may also help with housework if that is what is called for on a given day. The hours a doula works and her length of stay are variable, based on the needs of the particular family. Postpartum doulas are specifically trained to provide guidance and hands-on assistance during the postpartum period. See the Resources section in the back of the book for more information on finding a doula.

- *The Pet Sitter:* Many women are mothers to feline or canine children before having offspring of the human persuasion. Dogs in particular require a significant amount of attention between walks, grooming, and play time. Consider hiring a dog walker for the first few weeks to take some of the pressure off of needing to care for both Fido and your own offspring. Once you get into the groove, you can take everyone out for a nice walk around the block.

In countless ways, wonderful and sometimes bittersweet, bringing home a baby changes a couple's relationship. Where once there were two, now there are three and the ways in which a couple

Genuine interest in the other person unlocked the key to love in the beginning and it can do the same in entering this new stage of life together.

relates to each other and the world at large is forever changed. The family is different now and it can and should take some time to recalibrate and discover a new (and happy) normal.

After being coupled for some time, people tend to take for granted that partners know one another inside and out. There is an assumption that one individual can finish the other's sentences, that everything about the other is known. In reality, each person is a living organism, constantly growing and evolving. Becoming a parent requires a tremendous, holistic overhaul. Change is unavoidable. With this in mind, new parents should check in with each other, ask how the other is doing on a given day, even if they think they know the answer. Genuine interest in the other person unlocked the key to love in the beginning and it can do the same in entering this new stage of life together.

The idea behind *Mother Matters* is that every mother should be given access to effective, easy-to-learn, low- or no-cost tools that she may use to make the work of mothering easier to manage. Sometimes, though, even with every tool at one's disposal something more is needed. Sometimes a mom needs a boost beyond what she is able to do to care for herself and beyond what supportive friends and family may be able to give her. At some point during the course of the motherhood journey, many moms benefit from a play space of their own.

TALK IS *NOT* CHEAP

THE VALUE OF TALK THERAPY

When you don't talk, there's a lot of stuff
that ends up not getting said.

—Catherine Gilbert Murdock, American author

MAKING THE MONSTER DISAPPEAR:
AMELIA'S STORY

As a little girl, whenever I had a bad dream I would knock on my parents' bedroom door. My mother would rise from her bed, walk me back to my room, and gently tuck me back in. As she folded the blanket around my toes she would always say "Why don't you tell me about your dream? You'll feel better." I would tell her about the monster in my closet, the humongous shark *swimming around my school, or the creepy-crawly spiders taking over my bedroom walls. And then, like some sort of magic, I would fall back asleep without a worry. It was as if voicing the dream somehow destroyed the fear.*

Talking is among the most powerful antidotes to uncomfortable feelings—anxiety, sadness, and anger. Most people have the gift of speech, and when they are able to use it in partnership with a pair of listening ears, the result can be one of extraordinary healing.

Motherhood stirs up a wealth of emotion, often complicated to sort through on our own. Some feelings, like the joy of seeing baby's first smile, are right there on the surface. Others are more nuanced—more deeply buried—more difficult to process. The experience of having seemingly contradictory emotions from day to day, even moment to moment, is part of what makes the motherhood journey so rich and, at times, so intense.

Witnessing baby's first steps, for example, can elicit both pride and sadness; pride in the milestone baby has worked to reach and, perhaps, sadness at the reminder that these days are fleeting—baby is indeed growing up. One might even feel pleasure and despair at this fact alone—growth brings greater independence, which means less work for you, but it also underscores the reality of letting go, which every parent must learn to do if she wishes to help her child gain the autonomy necessary to move through the world.

From the time a woman is visibly pregnant, people—friends, family, and strangers—feel free to offer commentary. Some of their advice may be welcome. Some of it not. But nearly everyone has

> Most people have the gift of speech, and when they are able to use it in partnership with a pair of listening ears, the result can be one of extraordinary healing.

something to say about the status of motherhood. All of this chatter can drown out the singular voice that matters most—your own.

SECOND-GUESSING MY DECISION: TESSA'S STORY

I was out for a walk with my one-month-old. I had started taking her out for short walks in the stroller a week earlier. While I was anxious about keeping her comfortable—was she too warm or too cold, would she be hungry or cry before we returned—I remember feeling so free that we were able to be outside! My apartment was beginning to feel terribly claustrophobic. On the corner waiting for the traffic light to change, I lifted the blanket to check on Sasha who was sleeping peacefully. At that moment the woman standing next to me said, "What a beautiful baby! But she looks so little to be out and about." I wanted to slap her. And then I began to wonder if she was right. This stranger looked to be about my mom's age. Maybe she had raised children? Maybe she had more experience? Maybe she knew better than I? The joy I was feeling melted away and I was left wondering if I should just go back home.

Society sanctions the public sharing of opinions and judgments on certain subjects. Child-rearing is high atop the list. This is not meant to imply that others are consciously attempting to recruit each individual mom into their particular mother mindsets, but many people can't help but conflate their ways with the best ways.

What about those in your inner circle? Surrounding yourself with close friends and family, people who have had experience mothering and whose opinions are trusted can be comforting. However, whatever information is requested from these loved ones, whatever information is given, it is all filtered through the unique

Securing a safe and comfortable place to sort through all the comments, advice, and information in order to discover how you feel about it can be tremendously beneficial. lens of the giver. It may be colored by her personal history, your shared relationship, and where she is in her life physically and emotionally when the advice is offered. This is essential to keep in mind, especially when a mom is feeling vulnerable, which is often the case in the throes of the emotional upheaval and sleep deprivation characteristic of the newborn stage. At this time, securing a safe and comfortable place to sort through all the comments, advice, and information in order to discover how you feel about it can be tremendously beneficial. One way to do this is with a therapist.

FINDING MY OWN MOTHER-VOICE: BRIDGET'S STORY

I read just about every book on caring for a newborn by the time I had Andrew. I had taken infant CPR and massage classes and had learned about different positions for breastfeeding. I even started reading up on toddler beds to get ahead of the game. This is why what happened after I brought Andrew home from the hospital felt like such a shock to me! None of the breast-feeding positions I studied seemed to be working. Even though I bought the most highly recommended swaddling blanket on the market, he still managed to wriggle out of it. Every time I tried to calm his crying with a shushing sound it worked only for a few minutes and then he would be screaming again. Everything I did, even after all the planning, seemed to be a big fail. I felt exhausted and defeated. My mom friends had a lot to say, but they all said different things! And they couldn't really listen because they were busy with work or managing their own kids. I was at a loss for what to do and began feeling more and more confused and overwhelmed. My husband suggested it might help to talk to someone—a professional. At first, I was hurt and angry at the idea. "You don't think I can do this?!" I screamed at him. "You think I'm not cut out to be a mom!" One night, my husband brought home flowers and I nearly took his head off because finding a vase to put them in felt like too much effort. That was when he said, "Either you make an appointment or I'll make it for you." My ob-gyn gave me the name of a clinical social worker. I'll never forget our first session. The floodgates opened! I poured out all of the anxiety and uncertainty. She listened to me go on for forty-five minutes and didn't interrupt—not once. At the end of the session she thanked me for being so honest and courageous in sharing my feelings and said we might work well together. And we did. Talking to her has helped me find my voice. It has made me a better mother, a better partner, a better person.

There are many different kinds of talk therapy and many different styles of therapists, but the objective across the board should remain the same. A therapist should help you feel better. She or he should create a space in which you feel safe to explore deeply personal thoughts and feelings without judgment. The beauty of the therapeutic relationship is the freedom to be able to explore anything without fear of retribution or repercussions, as might be the case in the real world. You are in the driver's seat. A therapist is there to listen as you relay the events of your maternal journey—your life journey—and should be available to help you figure out where you are, where you want to go, and help guide you in figuring out how to get there.

An unfortunate misperception exists that therapy is somehow meant for those who are mentally ill or emotionally weak. Personal

There are many different kinds of talk therapy and many different styles of therapists, but the objective across the board should remain the same. A therapist should help you feel better.

and professional experience dictate that many people in therapy are quite the opposite—high functioning and well-adjusted. They may be, in fact, more psychologically healthy than the average Jane because they are consistent about putting in the work to maintain their own emotional welfare.

Exercise is a good analogy. If you go to the gym regularly and eat sensibly, you are more likely to continue to feel good and keep your body strong. Similarly, if you engage in a mental workout on a regular basis the same is likely to be true. Those first few workouts may be taxing if you are out of shape or have never exercised regularly, but once a routine is established, you may acquire and maintain a state of wellness that will enrich many aspects of your life.

For women who may have never been in therapy before, the onset of motherhood is a great time to start. For those who have been, this may be a good time to consider returning. Bringing home a baby is a high-stakes, all-hands-on-deck moment in a woman's life. She is entitled to all the support she can muster.

With that background, here's a primer on how to go about finding a therapist to help make life a little easier (after all, that's what life should be about right now, right?). The term *therapist* is an umbrella that covers a wide array of people with varying letters after their names, but doesn't offer much in the way of practical information. That's where the primer comes in.

For women who may have never been in therapy before, the onset of motherhood is a great time to start. For those who have been, this may be a good time to consider returning.

Read on to get the 411 on who can do what and where to find them.

THERAPY PRIMER: THE WHO'S WHO GLOSSARY

LICENSED CLINICAL SOCIAL WORKER (LCSW/LICSW)

An LCSW (or LICSW depending on where you live) is someone who holds a Masters in Social Work and has completed a number of years in the field providing clinical services, usually to a range of clientele. LCSWs are licensed by the state in which they practice and may work in a variety of settings from hospitals to social service agencies to schools. Many are in private practice. LCSWs may *not* prescribe medication, which is part of the reason why they are generally more affordable than other mental health practitioners, like psychiatrists. Often, they will have working relationships with colleagues who do have prescription-writing privileges and can make referrals when needed.

LICENSED MARRIAGE AND FAMILY THERAPIST (LMFT)

An LMFT is a state-licensed, Masters-level practitioner who typically focuses on treating couples or families as opposed to an individual. In the context of providing support to the client, in this case either the family-unit or the couple, an LMFT might meet with an individual on occasion. The bulk of the therapy though will include the couple or the family as a whole. LMFTs, like social workers, do not prescribe medication.

PSYCHIATRIC NURSE PRACTITIONER (NP)

There are many different kinds of nurse practitioners. Some specialize in general women's health, family, or pediatrics. Psychiatric nurse practitioners focus on mental health, and many do offer counseling. They work in a variety of healthcare environments from hospitals to private practice settings. While not physicians, they are able to write prescriptions.

PSYCHIATRIST

A psychiatrist is a medical doctor (MD) who specializes in working with patients who may have mental illness. In the old days before managed healthcare, psychiatrists had more of a reputation for offering talk therapy (you've heard of Sigmund Freud? He did that). These days, while some psychiatrists provide counseling, many others offer less talk and more medication. Often, a therapist such as an LCSW, will refer a client to a psychiatrist for medication management. In this case, the patient continues to see the LCSW for talk therapy and may briefly consult with the psychiatrist about a prescription (an antidepressant, for example) to enhance treatment.

Within the field of psychiatry, the practice of reproductive psychiatry has developed as a specialization. A reproductive psychiatrist specializes in women's mental health issues through the lifespan, and particularly those that relate to the menstrual cycle, menopause, and fertility.

PSYCHOLOGIST (PHD OR PSYD)

A psychologist is someone who has acquired a Masters or Doctoral degree and is licensed to practice. Psychology is a broad field and practitioners often specialize within a distinct area of psychology (clinical, industrial, school, environmental, etc.). Typically, a clinical psychologist would be the most likely of these to work with women during the postpartum period. Psychologists may hold a PhD (doctor of philosophy in psychology), but are not medical doctors and are thus not licensed to prescribe medication.

THE WHAT'S WHAT GLOSSARY: A BRIEF RUN-DOWN OF TALK THERAPIES

There are almost as many kinds of talk therapy as there are kinds of strollers. The purpose in including the following list is to provide a very basic understanding of some of the most commonly practiced forms. Some of them are more structured, others more fluid. Some are intended to be short-term, while others are ongoing. This very basic introduction includes information that may help you determine which kind of talk therapy and therapist might best resonate with you.

COGNITIVE BEHAVIORAL THERAPY (CBT)

CBT is a structured talk therapy that focuses on changing thoughts (cognitions) and behaviors. Through in-session exercises and between-session homework, CBT therapists help clients to change destructive thoughts and behaviors with the goal of lessening anxiety and other unpleasant emotions and increasing feelings of contentment. CBT has been proven very effective for treatment of conditions like Obsessive-Compulsive Disorder (OCD), which sometimes occurs for the first time during pregnancy or after birth. CBT is usually a time-limited therapy, meaning that a course of treatment generally lasts for a period of a few months, in contrast to other therapies that may continue indefinitely. One recent study evaluated the impact of a CBT group for women experiencing depressive symptoms in the first three months after childbirth. Moms met for six weekly two-hour group-sessions followed by a one-month follow-up session. At the conclusion, those who took part in CBT group experienced fewer symptoms than those in the control group, who did not (Mureşan Madar and Băban 2015, 51, 56).

EYE MOVEMENT DESENSITIZATION AND REPROCESSING (EMDR)

For moms who may have had the misfortune of a traumatic birth or who have a history of abuse, EMDR may be a smart option. Therapists who practice EMDR are specially trained in working with individuals who have experienced trauma, which, by the way, everyone has to varying degrees. While no one is sure exactly how it works, EMDR is a scientifically proven therapy that uses a non-invasive technique to help the brain reprocess traumatic experiences, making the disturbing material less upsetting and easier to manage. EMDR is also typically time-limited.

GROUP THERAPY

Therapy groups come in all different shapes and sizes (such as the CBT group described above). Here, the term is used loosely to include a wide range of group settings whose purpose is to provide support and education. New mom groups, commonly attended with baby in tow, offer an opportunity to meet other women transitioning to motherhood, share tips, and find camaraderie. Psychotherapy groups, by contrast, provide a forum to gain self-awareness in the company of others who are also interested in deeper insight. A friendly word of caution: A group can be a wonderful opportunity to connect and elevate your spirits, but only if it is the right group for you. Groups are most helpful when you feel safe and supported in sharing your feelings without fear of judgment. When this is the case, group therapy can work wonders.

PSYCHODYNAMIC PSYCHOTHERAPY

This style of treatment has its roots in psychoanalysis—Sigmund Freud's baby. But the method has come a long way since he was treating patients on the couch. Today, psychodynamic psycho-therapy may incorporate more than just what is happening in the unconscious. Personal history is used to inform how one operates in the present, which can be useful in figuring out why one mothers the way she does. The philosophy is that this knowledge can then help you to grow, evolve, and raise your level of awareness. This can lead to greater contentment. Psychodynamic psychotherapy is traditionally long-term, though financial and time constraints have made this less often the case in recent years. This modality may be a good choice for new mothers who experienced challenging childhoods themselves, including difficult relationships with their own parents.

TELETHERAPY

In the last few years, tele- and video therapy have been gaining in popularity. Apps like *Maven*, *Talkspace*, and *BetterHelp* allow users to browse different therapists, select one, and then schedule an online session at a mutually convenient time. For some people, the experience of connecting face-to-face with a therapist is more healing than talking through a smart phone or laptop. For others, the convenience of being able to access a sympathetic ear without leaving the house is a huge advantage.

If you are feeling severely depressed or are having thoughts of harming yourself or your baby, talk therapy is *not* an adequate solution. This should be considered an emergency and more immediate support is required. Speak with your doctor now. Serious postpartum or perinatal (in the time leading up to birth) depression is often entirely treatable and the sooner you take action to get the help you deserve, the more quickly you will begin to heal and feel better.

SO ... WHAT NOW?

Like a favorite pair of pre-pregnancy jeans, a therapist should be a comfortable fit. You may need to try a few on before deciding with whom to enter this unique relationship. In terms of where to start, there are a number of ways to go about finding someone:

HEALTH INSURANCE PROVIDER

Your health insurance company can provide a list of therapists who participate in your plan. These individuals should accept your insurance, making the cost of therapy significantly less than paying out-of-pocket. However, more and more therapists are opting not to take insurance because of the time-consuming paperwork, poor reimbursement, and other complexities that come with being on an insurance panel. If a therapist does not accept insurance, ask her if she offers a sliding scale—in which her fee may be adjusted depending on a client's financial position.

Like a favorite pair of pre-pregnancy jeans, a therapist should be a comfortable fit.

DOCTOR REFERRAL

Call your ob-gyn, midwife, general practitioner, or your baby's pediatrician and ask for a referral to a psychotherapist or support group in the area.

PSYCHOLOGYTODAY.COM

Enter your city and state of residence or zip code and a list of local mental healthcare providers will pop up.

FRIENDS AND FAMILY

Gal pals and cool Aunt Barb are wonderful for restaurant recommendations and other pearls of wisdom, but when it comes to something as crucial as your mental health, think twice about asking. Seeking out a referral from a friend or family member may open the door to questions and judgments—neither of which are likely to be beneficial. Please don't misunderstand; there is no shame or embarrassment in asking for help! On the contrary, the whole premise of this book is that help is a necessity at this time in life. The point here is simply that your business is just that—*your* business. If and with whom you choose to share it is entirely up to you.

Once you have a few names, it's time to check 'em out in person. Since time is at a premium, a couple of moments speaking on the phone with a few different providers is probably sufficient. Some questions to ask yourself as part of this due diligence: How do I feel on the phone with this person? Is she or he really listening? Do I get a good vibe? If you can answer a firm "yes" to these, that's a good place to start. Ask about bringing your baby to the session. Make a note both of the answer and of the tone of her response. Inquire about the fee and what forms of payment are accepted. Ultimately, when it comes to deciding on a therapist, turn down your intellectual voice and turn up your emotional one. Trust the gut—it usually knows before the head does.

Ultimately, when it comes to deciding on a therapist, turn down your intellectual voice and turn up your emotional one. Trust the gut—it usually knows before the head does.

A final note on therapy. Like many good things in life, it doesn't come easy and it doesn't come quick, but it can be well worth doing. In order for this tool to work, it requires a commitment. This is not to imply that you have to sign your life (or your bank account) away, but do be willing to do the following to maximize the potential benefits:

- Show up regularly for at least three months. Think of it as a fourth trimester. At that point, you and your therapist can evaluate how things are going.
- Do your homework in between sessions. If your therapist gives you an assignment, don't blow it off. Working on yourself between appointments can deepen the experience and sometimes expedite the effectiveness of treatment.
- Be honest. Lying to your therapist (and plenty of people do) only does you a disservice. If you don't feel you can trust this person, ask yourself why that might be. If the answer is compelling, find someone else.
- Be brave. Here's the thing about talk therapy: You may feel worse before you feel better. Not unlike birth itself, therapy can be painful, messy, and sometimes frightening. The result of going through this effort, though, can be beautiful, astonishing, and often positively life-changing.

Many new moms have found that spending some time in a therapist's office has made them feel a whole lot better. And for many moms, better feels pretty good.

MOTHERCARE, REALIZED

In giving birth to our babies, we may find that we
give birth to new possibilities within ourselves.

—Myla and Jon Kabat-Zinn, American authors

This is not a theoretical self-help guide. It is a practical one. The ideas explored here are concrete, accessible, and affordable.

Utilizing these resources can make a mother not only better able to fulfill her obligations to her child, but can make her much healthier and happier in the process.

Throughout the previous chapters, we have met mothers at a time when they needed a particular tool to help them manage a specific challenge within their maternal experience. In this final chapter, we will meet some moms whose postpartum phase was infused with greater relief, enjoyment, and personal growth as a direct result of identifying their needs and putting some of these tools into action.

The personal anecdotes that follow illustrate the ways moms like you have utilized this unique juncture in their lives to expand their own capabilities in ways they may have never imagined. I hope that they will inspire and encourage you to gain confidence in your own ability to seek and provide mothercare for yourself, as well as realize how doing so can transform your life.

NO APOLOGIES: LEAH'S STORY

Having my first child was a crash course in learning to ask for help. More than that, it was really about learning to ask for help unapologetically. I'm very organized and a hard worker—always have been. When Sam was born I realized, pretty quickly, that it was going to be impossible to operate in the way I was accustomed. I asked my sister if she could come over a few hours every week to watch Sam, and she generously agreed. As soon as she arrived each Wednesday afternoon, I high-tailed it out of my house. I didn't ask her how she was doing. I didn't make her a cup of coffee. I spent every last moment of those two hours on myself—taking a walk, getting my nails done, reading in the park, or meditating. If I was exhausted, I said a quick "hello and goodbye" and just went into my room and lay down. The purpose of this time was very clear—it was for me and me alone. I took full advantage of it, and I didn't apologize for doing so.

I also learned to say "no"—to everyone. "No, this is not a good time for you to drop by for a visit (but maybe next week)," "No, tomorrow morning won't work for a conference call (but I will get back to you with some other options)," "No, my love, I'm not in the mood right now (but I will be soon)." Lots of women struggle with saying "no." That isn't news. But, for the first time, becoming a mother enabled me to reframe how I feel about saying "no." Rather than believing I am in some way failing or letting someone else down, I now believe that saying "no" when I'm unable to commit to something whole-heartedly is really a generous act. It's a form of honesty, sincerity, and respect, both for myself and the other person. Saying "no" when I cannot, allows me to say "yes" authentically and eagerly when I can. I have carried these two lessons of early motherhood with me and they have served me very well in every area of my life.

On Sam's first birthday, I celebrated with a family party for him and a more intimate party for myself. I invested in a weekly babysitter and enrolled in a cooking class—French food! Learning to channel my inner Julia Child was on my bucket list, and this seemed like as good a time as any. Actually, it seemed like the perfect time. As he was growing up, I wanted to teach Sam how to eat mindfully and thoughtfully, and to feel a sense of gratitude for the food in front of him. Learning how to prepare a meal for my family felt like a natural extension of the mindful meditation practice I began after my son was born.

Sam turned three last week. He's doing great! And I'm still cookin'.

THE BIRTH OF A NEW PASSION: FATIMA'S STORY

My baby changed my life, sure, but not in the ways I imagined. It's like Shonda's birth triggered something in me or maybe planted a seed? I don't know. I don't really understand it, but I'm so grateful for it. I had been working in finance when she was born. After three months, I went back to the office. It was different. Not good or bad necessarily, just kind of—off. It's like it wasn't really my place anymore. I felt like I wanted to be working in another environment—to work with people in a more hands-on way—literally. I always loved massage therapy, and I saw the same masseuse for many years. After Shonda was born, I would bring her to my sessions, and she would treat us both, which was so much fun—we both felt so good afterwards. Having my daughter made me feel like it was now-or-never in terms of doing something I really felt passionate about. It was hard—no doubt. My husband had to be more available to take care of Shonda at night so

I could take classes. And it meant living on less. Our vacations don't look the same as they used to. A massage therapist doesn't make the same salary as a VP in finance—ha!—not even in the same ballpark. But I haven't looked back. I love how I spend my days now. I love working with women in particular—offering them some relief from their everyday stressors. Something opened up for me when Shonda was born; beyond becoming her mama, I became more of myself.

My daughter is eighteen months old now. Sometimes I think about the woman I was before I gave birth to her and the woman I am now. I'm thankful that she is getting to know this version of me—it's a better one. Having a baby is stressful, but in a weird way, becoming a mom has actually made me less stressed. Well, maybe not less stressed, but it has made me better able to manage my stress. My daughter gave me a real gift in that way. She taught me that I could—that I should—do something I love to do—that feels right. I realize how lucky I am to be able to do it—and I'm so grateful. My wish for her is that she learns from a very early age that her feelings matter—that her well-being matters. I want her to learn to take care of herself as a girl so that she will carry those habits with her throughout her life. And I feel like part of my job as her mom is to model that for her.

As for me, I feel like becoming a massage therapist is the beginning of my own journey, not the final destination. The more I learn, the more I want to learn. There are so many healing techniques that have come up while I've been studying that I'm curious about. Shiatsu, Reiki, Thai massage—there are so many directions I can go in and that's really exciting.

COMING INTO MY BODY: SHARI'S STORY

For me, one of the most amazing things about becoming a mother was the way it changed my relationship with my body. I was lucky in that I had a pretty easy pregnancy. The first trimester was kind of rough—I was really nauseous for most of it; but after those three months, it eased up and my energy returned. I took a prenatal yoga class, which helped me better understand what was happening in my body and helped prepare me for labor and delivery. Once I met my gorgeous Alexander, I was just kind of in awe about what my body was able to do. I wanted other women to feel that way, too. There is so much body-shaming for us—so much comparing of ourselves to others and trying to be perfect. I continued taking yoga classes even after Alex started school. I also started jogging a couple of times a week with a mom friend. I always heard about the pressure to lose the baby weight and the race to get back to that pre-pregnancy body. For me, though, I just felt like Superwoman after I had my son. Whenever I felt tired or under the weather after that, I tried to remember what my body was capable of doing and it helped me through. I also felt more dedicated to keeping it healthy and strong; my body had given me the gift of my child, and I wanted to give it something back.

Alexander is three years old now, and guess what . . . I just found out I'm pregnant—seven weeks! I know every pregnancy is different, just like every child is, but I hope that the attitude I have toward my body now will help keep me feeling good. Actually, a friend of mine said that acupressure really helped her morning sickness, so I am going to give it a try—and maybe even acupuncture to help with labor pain, too. I guess I have some time to decide on that one!

HAVING MORE FUN: JILL'S STORY

I was just so tired those first couple of months. The lack of sleep was brutal. I thought that once Mason started sleeping through the night (around four months, I think), I would start to feel better. Don't get me wrong, I loved being able to sleep more, but to be honest, my brain just started to get mushy. Did anyone ever die from boredom? I had this moment of reckoning when I realized I didn't like being a mom. It was kind of awful. I mean, I loved Mason more than any-thing, but I just remember craving something new and different—an activity to kind of spice up our days—at least something I could do to talk with my partner about at the end of the day. For me, joining a mother-infant art class was amazing. I loved being able to be creative and make something new. And I loved that I could make this one mess and not have to clean it up!

Even though the class only met once a week, sometimes I would bring home a project to work on at night or when Mason was tak-ing a nap. It just tapped into a different part of my brain than that part responsible for feeding, changing, and general baby care. And I loved that. Art-making was never something I would have even considered before my daughter was born, but now I feel like it is a part of who I am. I've noticed, too, that the creativity I bring to my art helps me in work, too. As a high school social studies teacher, I'm always looking for new and interesting ways to engage my class. I've started bringing in art work to the room—sometimes a piece that was made during the time period we are studying or one that is rel-evant to the subject we are learning about. It doesn't always work, obviously, but often it gets the kids talking and sometimes it sparks a really interesting conversation.

Mason is two years old now and let me tell you, the terrible twos are no joke. She is a force to be reckoned with! I'm scared to see what the teenage years will bring, but whatever happens, I feel like I can handle it. As long as I remember to come back to being creative—it's like my fuel. It gives me the emotional bandwidth to manage when things seem hard. And that feels really empowering.

DISCOVERING A DEEPER PART OF ME: STELLA'S STORY

I was (mostly) prepared for what the newborn experience would be like. As the oldest of five, taking care of my younger brothers and sisters was a big part of my own childhood. I didn't mind it really. I enjoyed helping my mom out and it made me feel kind of important in the family. Maybe for all of these reasons, I was surprised by my feelings when I had my own child. I was the first of my siblings to have a baby, so I couldn't really ask them for advice. My mom would help when I asked her, but she never really offered to help. I wondered if maybe she was just sort of worn out after raising her own kids for so many years. I mean, it made sense, but it also made me so angry! She made me feel guilty when I asked her for a hand. She would say things like, "Well, I can come over, but I have to reschedule my bridge game." Ugh! It drove me crazy. I was so tired and stressed out that I started snapping at my husband, and I was more and more impatient with my daughter. A friend of mine was a therapist and thought it might help me to see someone. I put it off for a while. I just wasn't sure I wanted to delve into all that baggage. Eventually, though, the thought of talking through my feelings with someone was less scary than the realization that I was not the person I wanted to be. My therapist helped me more than I can say. It was hard, and it was painful sometimes. But I learned so much about myself and about my relationship with my own mom. More than that, I learned how to share my feelings in a way that was productive, and that changed our relationship for the better. Actually, it changed many of my relationships for the better. I feel much more confident in my ability to build a healthy connection with my own daughter because of the work I have done on myself.

Alexis is four now. She is very close with her "Nay-Nay," and I like to think that this is at least in part because of the work I did to make it so. Working with my therapist, which I still do to this day, is not a luxury for me. It is part of an overall commitment I make to take care of me, just as I take care of my daughter, my husband, and others in my family.

I think maybe the biggest thing I learned when I became a mom, although it continues to be a work in progress, is that my well-being is not an option. I think maybe that was part of the difference between me and my own mother. She never really learned to take care of herself. She was not encouraged to do so. With each child she had, the demands increased, but the ability to meet them didn't. I think if she had been in an environment that recognized mothers need help and made it readily available to them—without judgment—things might have looked very different growing up.

Though the details of these stories differ, a singular thread unites them. These women seized their own transitions to motherhood to probe more deeply into themselves. They used this time to focus on their own well-being: to discover, empower, and become more authentic and contented. They did so by recognizing their own value and the need to preserve and protect this precious commodity. In some cases, they needed to make adjustments in their lives in order to enable their growth. Fatima took a big pay cut. Jill bravely acknowledged that she needed something beyond the work of daily mothering to find fulfillment and Stella went through an emotional, at times deeply painful, journey in counseling.

As all of them agree, though, the results of their efforts paid off in big dividends and will continue to do so well into the future.

There is nothing these women have that you do not. You have everything needed, right now, to honor your mother self. When you are ready, I invite you to share your own story at daynamkurtz .com. In so doing, you will inspire others toward the mothercare movement. Together, we will make it a reality.

Remember always that the effort involved in raising a happy, healthy child is immeasurable. So, too, are the rewards. As children mature and the sounds of daily mothering shift from a roar to a whisper, know that the tools in this book may be used at any time, at any age, at any stage. After all, whatever the point in time, mothers always matter.

TEMPLATES

MOOD LOG (EXAMPLE)

Date	Time of day	Feeling before exercise	Exercise (activity & duration)	Feeling after exercise	Baby present?
April 12	11:15 am	Sluggish	Walk, 30 minutes	More energized	N
April 15	2:30 pm	Content	Watch, Wait & Wonder, 20 minutes	Curious	Y

MOOD LOG

Date	Time of day	Feeling before exercise	Exercise (activity & duration)	Feeling after exercise	Baby present?

FOOD JOURNAL (EXAMPLE)

Date	Time of day	I'm feeling ... because ...	Craving	Choice
September 9	1:30 pm	Tired because baby skipped her morning nap	Potato chips	I will count out 20 chips and put the bag away.
September 12	11:00 am	Sad because ... I'm not sure ...	Cookies	I will go for a walk instead.

FOOD JOURNAL

Date	Time of day	I'm feeling ... because ...	Craving	Choice

ACKNOWLEDGEMENTS

MOTHERS MATTER, AND SO DO the people who love and support them. I am blessed to be surrounded by a remarkably kind, generous, and wise group of relatives, friends, and colleagues. Those named here have been integral players in the delivery of this book.

Thank you to Diane Stockwell, my agent at Globo Libros Literary Management, for taking a chance on a first-time author.

To my entire Familius family: Christopher, Brooke, David, Erika, and my editor extraordinaire (and mother of nine, I might add) Michele. Thank you all for believing both in the message of *Mother Matters* and for providing the opportunity to share it with new moms (and dads) everywhere.

Setting out to write a book can be an overwhelming endeavor. Surrounding oneself with those familiar with this oft lonely and sometimes arduous task, and generous enough to commiserate and share guidance, greatly eases the burden. Thank you to fellow writers Doug Most, Tina Cassidy, Annmarie Kelly-Harbaugh, and Lisa Sugarman.

My sincere gratitude to Karen Starr, for her gentle and insightful mentorship as I crafted early drafts of this book, and to Amy Weber, Chaim Bromberg, and Hannah Hahn for their thoughtful reading and supportive critique, which helped make those drafts better.

I expected that researching the tools contained herein would be enlightening. I was pleasantly surprised when it turned out also to be joyous. This was due in large part to the fact that the experts with whom I consulted are not only supremely knowledgeable in their chosen disciplines, but are also incredibly thoughtful people. They shared their insight with great eagerness and clarity, and they were always readily available to answer additional questions as they arose. Connecting with them in this pursuit has been a deep privilege. Thank you to Ashley Flores, Amanda Tarver, Mary Jane Detroyer, Cassandra Hall Primeau, and Kaeli Macdonald.

Many thanks also to the researchers, educators, and clinicians, too many to name, whose invaluable contributions to the wealth of studies on maternal and infant health profoundly informed this writing and affirmed my faith that the mothercare movement is indeed possible.

Valerie Conlan and David Horvath told me I should write a book. Perhaps more importantly, they encouraged me to finish it. They are among the most big-hearted people I know, and I love them dearly.

Patricia Gilroy designed the meal plan contained herein and shared much of the included dietary suggestions. Patricia and I met as a result of our children when we found ourselves in a very special playgroup together. She is a remarkable mother to three boys and an inspiring woman in her own right. I am grateful for her friendship.

To the late Alice Rosenman and to Joan Musitano, who facilitated that very special aforementioned playgroup and in so doing, co-created an invaluable resource as I maneuvered through the earliest days of my own maternal transition.

My deep thanks to the remarkable people at The School of Practical Philosophy in New York City. I am fortunate enough to be a student at this unique place of learning, which provides access to concrete tools for living in a more meaningful, peaceful, and connected way. My classmates and tutors have made me a better writer and (I hope) a better person.

My friends—some mothers, others not, but all believers in mothercare—have been hugely supportive during my book's gestation. They have pulled me away from my laptop when I needed it and pushed me toward it when I needed that, too. Very special thanks to the remarkable Kate Cosgriff, Elizabeth Brown, Marina Vytovtova, Heather Church, Alanna Yudin, Robin Broshi, Rachel Breitman, Paula Clarkson, Rebekah Heusel, Annie Stone, Marci Kaplan, Beth Satlin, Brett Douglas, Ayala Cohen, Maris Pasquale Doran, Josie Torielli, and John McCaffrey.

Many thanks to my in-laws, Carol and Michael Kurtz and Randy and Lauren Kurtz, and also to my brother, Adam Steinfeld, and sister-in-law, Stacy Rothrock-Steinfeld, for their consistent support and encouragement and for asking all the right questions.

To Alan and Rena Steinfeld: The world would be a far better place if every child was gifted with the kind of parents that mine are to me. They are the sort who make a child feel she can succeed in every endeavor and the first ones there to help her back on her feet when she inevitably does not. Quite simply, they created a foundation by which writing this book became not only possible, but actual. From being available to babysit (often at a moment's notice), to reading excerpts, to brainstorming, to networking, to cheerleading, they stepped in to fulfill whatever need popped up, whenever it popped up. Beyond all of this, they are simply wonderful people, the kind I would choose to spend time with voluntarily. In fact, I do. If you ever had the opportunity to do the same, I strongly encourage it. Thank you, Mom and Dad. I love you.

Last, and a world away from least, I want to thank my husband, Jason. A full-time psychotherapist and part-time playwright, he is a wonder to behold. When we were dating and things got serious,

I shored up my courage and told him I wasn't sure I wanted children, fearing this might be a deal-breaker. His response? "I want *you*. The rest will sort itself." Lucky for me, we've been sorting together ever since.

Jason, you are my sounding board, my moral compass, my partner in work, in play, and in parenting. Your influence permeates the pages of this book. Thank you for loving me and for always making me feel that I matter.

RESOURCES

Some of the resources listed below do not cater specifically to new mothers. When searching for an individual practitioner (like a massage or art therapist, for example), be sure that the person has additional training in working with postnatal clients.

ACUPUNCTURE & ACUPRESSURE

- National Certification Commission for Acupuncture and Oriental Medicine: mx.nccaom.org/FindAPractitioner
- Australian Acupuncture and Chinese Medicine Association: acupuncture.org.au
- The Chinese Medicine and Acupuncture Association of Canada: cmaac.ca
- British Acupuncture Council: acupuncture.org.uk
- Acupressure is not currently a licensed discipline. Look for a practitioner who is licensed in massage therapy and has an additional certification in acupressure here: therubhub.com/acupressure-listing_subcategory-58.php

COUNSELING, THERAPY & MATERNAL MENTAL HEALTH

- Psychology Today (offers a "find a local therapist" feature): psychologytoday.com

- Postpartum Support International: postpartum.net
- American Association for Marriage and Family Therapy (offers a "find a local therapist" feature): aamft.org
- Canadian Counselling and Psychotherapy Association: ccpa-accp.ca
- Psychotherapy and Counselling Federation of Australia: pacfa.org.au
- Mental Health Foundation (UK): mentalhealth.org.uk

DOULA CARE

- DONA International: dona.org

EXERCISE

- Daynamkurtz.com
- Strollercize: strollercize.com
- Fit4Mom: Fit4Mom.com
- Pronatal Fitness: pronatalfitness.com

EXPRESSIVE-ARTS THERAPY

- American Art Therapy Association: arttherapy.org
- Canadian Art Therapy Association: canadianarttherapy .org
- Australian Creative Arts Therapies Association: acata .org.au
- The British Association of Art Therapists: baat.org

HEALTHFUL EATING & EATING DISORDERS

- Academy of Nutrition and Dietetics: eatright.org/ find-an-expert

- National Eating Disorders Association: nationaleating disorders.org
- National Eating Disorder Information Centre (Canada): nedic.ca
- The Nutrition Society of Australia: nsa.asn.au
- British Association for Applied Nutrition & Nutritional Therapy: bant.org.uk

MASSAGE

- American Massage Therapy Association: amtamassage .org/findamassage/index.html
- "Infant Massage—Relax Baby and Relieve Colic Full Compilation," featuring Susan Salvo, youtube.com/ watch?v=NqR_YkYYw54
- "Baby 101: How To Massage Your Infant," featuring Brandi Jordan, youtube.com/watch?v=rrASOAFRf-s
- International Association of Infant Massage: iaim.net

MEDITATION & MINDFULNESS

- Jon Kabat-Zinn, PhD: mindfulnesscds.com
- Amy Saltzman, MD: stillquietplace.com
- Carla Naumburg, PhD: carlanaumburg.com
- Cassandra Vieten, PhD, audio meditation: library.noetic.org/library/audio-experientials/ mindful-awareness-breathing-meditation
- Kripalu Center for Yoga & Health: kripalu.org
- Vipassana Meditation: dhamma.org/en-US/index

REFERENCES

INTRODUCTION

Page	*Note*

2   Winnicott, D. W. (1971). *Playing and reality.* Middlesex, England: Penguin Books Ltd. p. 163.

3   Winnicott, D. W. (1953). Transitional objects and transitional phenomena—a study of the first not-me possession. *International Journal of Psychoanalysis, 34,* 89–97. Retrieved from http://onlinelibrary.wiley .com/journal/10.1111/(ISSN)1745-8315.

3   Winnicott, D. W. (1971). *Playing and reality.* Middlesex, England: Penguin Books Ltd.

3   Benjamin, J. (1995). Recognition and destruction: An outline of intersubjectivity. In J. Benjamin, *Like Subjects, Love Objects: Essays on Recognition and Sexual Difference.* New Haven, CT: Yale University Press.

3   Ibid. p. 42.

CHILDCARE. ELDERCARE. MOTHERCARE? WHAT'S *MOTHERCARE?*

7   King, T. (2013). The mismatch between postpartum services and women's needs: Supermom versus lying-in. *Journal of Midwifery & Women's Health, 58*(6), 607. doi:10.1111/jmwh.12138

12   Douglas, S. J., and Michaels, M. W. (2004). *The Mommy Myth: The Idealization of Motherhood and How It Has Undermined All Women.* New York: Free Press.

12   Winnicott, D. W. (1971). *Playing and reality.* Middlesex, England: Penguin Books Ltd.

15   Doss, B. D., Rhoades, G. K., Stanley, S. M., and Markman, H. J. (March 2009). The effect of the transition to parenthood on relationship quality: An 8-year prospective study. *Journal of Personality and Social Psychology, 96*(3), 601–619. doi:10.1037/a0013969

ACUPUNCTURE & ACUPRESSURE: THE BENEFITS OF PINS & NEEDLES

19–20   Birch, S. (2015). Understanding Qi in clinical practice—perspectives from an acupuncture scholar-practitioner. *Journal of Chinese Medicine, 107,* 58–63.

20   Samadi, D. (May 15, 2012). More Americans using acupuncture for common ailments. *Fox News.* Retrieved from http://www.foxnews.com/health/2012/05/15/more-americans-using-acupuncture-for-common-ailments.html.

20   Battaloğlu Inanç, B. (2015). A new theory on the evaluation of traditional Chinese acupuncture mechanisms from the latest medical scientific point of view. *Acupuncture & Electro-Therapeutics Research, 40*(3), 189–204.

20   White, A., and Editorial Board of Acupuncture in Medicine. (2009). Western medical acupuncture: a definition. *Acupuncture in Medicine, 27*(1), 33–5. doi: 10.1136/aim.2008.000372

20   Zhao, Y., and Guo, H. (2006). The therapeutic effects of acupuncture in 30 cases of postpartum hypogalactia. *Journal of Traditional Chinese Medicine, 26*(1), 29–30.

22   Jimenez, S. (1995). Acupressure: Pain relief at your fingertips. *International Journal of Childbirth Education, 10*(4), 7–10.

23   Kuo, S. Y., Tsai, S. H., Chen, S. L., and Tzeng, Y. L. (2016). Auricular acupressure relieves anxiety and fatigue, and reduces cortisol levels in post-Caesarean section women: A single-blind, randomised controlled study. *International Journal of Nursing Studies, 53*, 17–26. doi:10.1016/j.ijnurstu.2015.10.006

23   Esfahani, M. S., Berenji-Sooghe, S., Valiani, M., and Ehsanpour, S. (2015). Effect of acupressure on milk volume of breastfeeding mothers referring to selected health care centers in Tehran. *Iranian Journal of Nursing & Midwifery Research, 20*(1), 7–11.

31–32   Jimenez, S. (1995). Acupressure: Pain relief at your fingertips. *International Journal of Childbirth Education, 10*(4), 7–10.

32   Flores, A., Skype interview, February 11, 2016.

EXPRESSIVE-ARTS THERAPY: MORE THAN ARTS & CRAFTS

36   Hosea, H. (2006). "The Brush's Footmarks": Parents and infants paint together in a small community art therapy group. *International Journal of Art Therapy, 11*(2), 69–78. doi:10.1080/17454830600980317

36   Snir, S., and Regev, D. (2013). A dialog with five art materials: Creators share their art making experiences. *The Arts in Psychotherapy, 40,* 94–100. doi:10.1016/j.aip.2012.11.004

36   Perry, C., Thurston, M., and Osborn, T. (2008). Time for Me: The arts as therapy in postnatal depression. *Complementary Therapies in Clinical Practice, 14*(1), 38–45. doi:10.1016/j.ctcp.2007.06.001

36   Arroyo, C., and Fowler, N. (2013). Before and after: A mother infant painting group. *International Journal of Art Therapy, 18*(3), 98–112.

36   Macdonald, K., Skype interview, February 15, 2016.

37   Ibid.

38   American Art Therapy Association. What is art therapy. Retrieved from http://arttherapy.org/aata -aboutus.

38   Hosea, H. (2006). "The Brush's Footmarks": Parents and infants paint together in a small community art therapy group. *International Journal of Art Therapy, 11*(2), 69–78. doi:10.1080/17454830600980317

39   Winnicott, D. W. (1971). *Playing and reality.* Middlesex, England: Penguin Books Ltd.

40   Arroyo, C., and Fowler, N. (2013). Before and after: A mother infant painting group. *International Journal of Art Therapy, 18*(3), 102.

41   Ibid. pp. 98–112.

41   Perry, C., Thurston, M., and Osborn, T. (2008). Time for Me: The arts as therapy in postnatal depression. *Complementary Therapies in Clinical Practice, 14*(1), 38–45. doi:10.1016/j.ctcp.2007.06.001

43   Macdonald, K., Skype interview, February 15, 2016.

44   Ibid.

47   Fitzpatrick, K. (August 1, 2017). Why adult coloring books are good for you. *CNN.* Retrieved from http://www.cnn.com/2016/01/06/health/adult-coloring-books-popularity-mental-health/index.html.

FEED ME! HEALING MEALS FOR MAMAS

52   Kolata, G. (May 2, 2016). After "The Biggest Loser," their bodies fought to regain weight. *New York Times.* Retrieved from https://www.nytimes.com/2016/05/02/health/biggest-loser-weight-loss.html.

54   Hart, J. (2014). Healthy behaviors linked to practice of mindful eating. *Alternative & Complementary Therapies, 20*(6), 317–319. doi:10.1089/act.2014.20605

54   Warriner, S., Dymond, M., and Williams, M. (2013). Mindfulness in maternity. *British Journal of Midwifery, 21*(7), 520–522.

57   Detroyer, M. J., Skype interview, May 15, 2016.

59   Gilroy, P., email interview, June 9, 2016.

59   Ibid.

60   Scholey, A., and Owen, L. (2013). Effects of chocolate on cognitive function and mood: A systematic review. *Nutrition Reviews, 71*(10), 665–681.

62   Cox, A. (February 6, 2017). When can I start giving my baby peanut butter? American Academy of Pediatrics. Retrieved from https://www.healthychildren.org /English/tips-tools/ask-the-pediatrician/Pages /When-can-I-start-giving-my-baby-peanut-butter .aspx.

63   Taylor, M. (January 14, 2017). 8 cleanest, healthiest frozen entrées you can buy. Prevention. Retrieved from www.prevention.com/eatclean /clean-frozen-entrees.

63   Carroll, A. E. (May 23, 2016). Sorry, there's nothing magical about breakfast. *New York Times.* Retrieved from http://www.nytimes.com/2016/05/24/upshot /sorry-theres-nothing-magical-about-breakfast.html.

MEAL PLANNER GUIDE

67   Gilroy, P., email interviews, June 9–September 27, 2016.

77   Etebary, S. et al. (2010.) Postpartum depression and role of serum trace elements. *Iranian Journal of Psychiatry, 5*(2), 40–46.

FLEXERCISE: HOW A LITTLE WORKOUT CAN GO A LONG WAY

84   Van Dusen, A. (February 2008). Ten reasons you're a couch potato. Retrieved November 13, 2016, from http://www.forbes.com/2008/02/27/health-couch -exercise-forbeslife-cx_avd_0227potato.html.

85   Dunn, A. L., and Jewell, J. S. (2010). The effect of exercise on mental health [abstract]. *Current Sports Medicine Reports, 9*(4), 202–7. Retrieved from http:// www.ncbi.nlm.nih.gov/pubmed/20622537.

85   Currie, J., and Develin, E. (2002). Stroll your way to well-being. A survey of the perceived benefits, barriers, community support, and stigma associated with pram walking groups designed for new mothers, Sydney, Australia. *Health Care For Women International, 23,* 882–93. Retrieved from http:// www.tandfonline.com/toc/uhcw20/current.

85   Bandura, A. (1994). Self-efficacy. In V. S. Ramachaudran (Ed.), *Encyclopedia of Human Behavior* (Vol. 4, pp. 71–81). New York: Academic Press.

(Reprinted in H. Friedman [Ed.], *Encyclopedia of Mental Health.* San Diego: Academic Press, 1998.)

86   Shorey, S., Chan, S. W., Chong, Y. S., and He, H. G. (2015). Predictors of maternal parental self-efficacy among primiparas in the early postnatal period. *Western Journal of Nursing Research, 37*(12), 1604–22. doi:10.1177/0193945914537724

86   LeCheminant, J. D., Hinman, T., Pratt, K. B., Earl, N., Bailey, B. W., Thackeray, R., and Tucker, L. A. (2014). Effect of resistance training on body composition, self-efficacy, depression, and activity in postpartum women. *Scandinavian Journal of Medicine & Science in Sports, 24,* 414–21. doi:10.111 1/j.1600-0838.2012.01490

86   Jackson, D. (2010). How personal trainers can use self-efficacy theory to enhance exercise behavior in beginning exercisers. *Strength and Conditioning Journal, 32*(3), 67–71. doi:10.1519 /SSC.0b013e3181d81c10

86   David, R. L., and Butki, B. D. (1998). Self-efficacy and affective responses to short bouts of exercise. *Journal of Applied Sport Psychology, 10*(2), 268–80. doi:10.1080/10413209808406393

86   Carey, G. B., Quinn, T. J., and Goodwin, S. E. (1997). Breast milk composition after exercise of different intensities. *Journal of Human Lactation, 13*(2), 115–20. Retrieved from http://jhl.sagepub.com.

87   Mortensen, K., and Kam, R. (2012). Exercise and breastfeeding. *Breastfeeding Review, 20*(3), 39–42.

Retrieved from https://www.breastfeeding.asn.au /bfreview.

87 Lovelady, C., Bopp, M., Colleran, H., Mackie, H., and Wideman, L. (2009). Effect of exercise training on loss of bone mineral density during lactation. *Medicine & Science in Sports & Exercise, 41*(10), 1902–7. Retrieved from http://ezproxy.library.nyu .edu:2079/10.1249/MSS.0b013e3181a5a68b.

87 American Heart Association. Facts about heart disease in women. Retrieved from https://www.go redforwomen.org/home/about-heart-disease-in -women/facts-about-heart-disease.

87 Spratling, P., Pryor, E., Moneyham, L., Hodges, A., White-Williams, C., and Martin, J. Jr. (2014). Effect of an educational intervention on cardiovascular disease risk perception among women with preeclampsia. *Journal of Obstetric, Gynecologic & Neonatal Nursing, 43*, 179–89. doi:10.1111/1552-6909.12296

87 Fadl, H., Magnuson, A., Ostlund, I., Montgomery, S., and Schwarcz, E. (2014). Gestational diabetes mellitus and later cardiovascular disease: A Swedish population based case-control study. *British Journal of Obstetrics and Gynecology, 121*, 1530–36. Retrieved from http://www.bjog.org/view/0/index.html.

87–88 Carpenter, R. E., Emery, S. J., Uzun, O., D'Silva, L. A., and Lewis, M. J. (2015). "Influence of antenatal physical exercise on haemodynamics in pregnant women: a flexible randomisation approach." *BMC Pregnancy & Childbirth, 15*(1), 1–15. doi:10.1186/ s12884-015-0620-2

88   Dritsa, M., Da Costa, D., Dupuis, G., Lowensteyn, I., and Khalifé, S. (2008). "Effects of a home-based exercise intervention on fatigue in postpartum depressed women: results of a randomized controlled trial." *Annals of Behavioral Medicine: A Publication of the Society of Behavioral Medicine*, 35(2), 179–87. doi:10.1007/s12160-008-9020-4

88   Ashrafinia, F., Mirmohammadali, M., Rajabi, H., Kazemnejad, A., Haghighi, K.S., and Amelvalizadeh, M. (2015). "Effect of Pilates exercises on postpartum maternal fatigue." *Singapore Medical Journal*, 56(3), 169–73. doi:10.11622/smedj.2015042

89   American College of Sports Medicine. (2013). ACSM information on resistance training for health and fitness. Retrieved November 13, 2016, from https://www.acsm.org/docs/default-source/brochures/resistance-training.pdf?sfvrsn=6.

89   The Centers for Disease Control and Prevention. Current physical activity guidelines. Retrieved November 26, 2017, from https://www.cdc.gov/cancer/dcpc/prevention/policies_practices/physical_activity/guidelines.htm.

90   Hydration while breastfeeding. Ask Dr. Sears. Retrieved from http://www.askdrsears.com/topics/feeding-eating/breastfeeding/hydration-while-breastfeeding.

92   Daley, A., MacArthur, C., and Winter, H. (2007). The role of exercise in treating postpartum depression: A review of the literature. *Journal of Midwifery*

and Women's Health, 52(1), 56–62. doi:10.1016 /j.jmwh.2006.08.017

93   Currie, J., and Develin, E. (2002). Stroll your way to well-being. A survey of the perceived benefits, barriers, community support, and stigma associated with pram walking groups designed for new mothers, Sydney, Australia. *Health Care for Women International, 23,* 882–93.

93   Targum, S. D., and Rosenthal, N. (2008). Seasonal affective disorder. *Psychiatry (Edgmont), 5*(5), 31–33. Retrieved from http://www.ncbi.nlm.nih.gov/pmc /articles/PMC2686645.

98   American College of Sports Medicine. (2013). Resistance training for health and fitness. Retrieved from www.acsm.org/docs/brochures/resistance -training.pdf.

99   American College of Sports Medicine. ACSM issues new recommendations on quantity and quality of exercise. Retrieved from http://www.acsm.org /about-acsm/media-room/news-releases/2011/08/01 /acsm-issues-new-recommendations-on-quantity -and-quality-of-exercise.

104–5 Boissonnault, J. S., and Blaschak M. J. (1988). Incidence of diastasis recti abdominis during the childbearing year. *Physical Therapy, 68*(7), 1082–6. Retrieved from http://ptjournal.apta.org /?navID=10737423605.

107   Maechler, A. (2013). Clubs can tap into growth of Pilates and yoga with dedicated studios. *Club*

Industry, 29(10), 18–20. Retrieved from clubindustry .com.

108 Ko, Y., Yang, C., Fang, C., Lee, M., and Lin, P. (2013). Community-based postpartum exercise program. *Journal of Clinical Nursing, 22*(15/16), 2122–31. doi: 10.1111/jocn.12117

108 Ashrafinia, F., Mirmohammadali, M., Rajabi, H., Kazemnejad, A., Sadeghniiat Haghighi, K., and Amelvalizadeh, M. (2015). Effect of Pilates exercises on postpartum maternal fatigue. *Singapore Medical Journal, 56*(3), 169–73. doi:10.11622/smedj.2015042

MATERNAL MASSAGE THERAPY: HANDS-ON HEALING

111–12 Deligiannidis, K. M., and Freeman, M. P. (2014). Complementary and alternative medicine therapies for perinatal depression. *Best Practice & Research: Clinical Obstetrics & Gynaecology, 28*(1), 85–95.

112 Fadzil, F., Shamsuddin, K., and Wan Puteh, S. E. (2016). Traditional postpartum practices among Malaysian mothers: A review. *Journal of Alternative and Complementary Medicine, 22*(7), 503–508. doi:10.1089/acm.2013.0469

112 Hall, G. H., Griffiths, D. L., and McKenna, L. G. (2011). The use of complementary and alternative medicine by pregnant women: A literature review. *Midwifery, 27*(6), 817–24. doi:10.1016/j.midw.2010.08.007

114 Tarver, A., email interview, August 22–23, 2016.

116   Ko, Y., and Lee, H. (2014). Randomised controlled trial of the effectiveness of using back massage to improve sleep quality among Taiwanese insomnia postpartum women. *Midwifery, 30*(1), 60–64. Retrieved from http://www.midwiferyjournal .com/article/S0266-6138(12)00211-2/fulltext.

116   American Pregnancy Association. (2015). Postpartum massage. Retrieved from http://americanpregnancy .org/first-year-of-life/postpartum-massage.

117   Tarver, A., email interview, August 22–23, 2016.

118   Choi, M. S., and Lee, E. J. (2015). Effects of foot-reflexology massage on fatigue, stress and postpartum depression in postpartum women. *Journal of Korean Academy of Nursing, 45*(4), 587–94. doi:10.4040 /jkan.2015.45.4.587

118   Imura, M., Misao, H., and Ushijima, H. (2006). The psychological effects of aromatherapy-massage in healthy postpartum mothers. *The Journal of Midwifery & Women's Health, 51*, 21–27. doi:10.1016 /j.jmwh.2005.08.009

119   Hall Primeau, C., email interview, August 24, 2016.

122   Cooke, A. (2015). Infant massage: The practice and evidence-base to support it. *British Journal of Midwifery, 23*(3). doi:http://dx.doi.org/10.12968 /bjom.2015.23.3.166

123   Infant Massage USA. (2016). Asking permission. Retrieved from http://infantmassageusa.org/parents /parents.php#askingpermission.

124   Ibid.

125   Salvo, S. (September 16, 2013). *Infant massage—relax baby & relieve colic.* Retrieved from https://www.youtube.com/watch?v=jjiQMf77kGY.

125   McClure, V. (2017). *Infant Massage: A Handbook for Loving Parents* (4th rev. ed.). New York: Bantam Books, p. 147.

125   Salvo, S. Infant Massage—Relax Baby and Relieve Colic Full Compilation. YouTube video, 10:15, from an instructional demonstration posted January 20, 2017, https://www.youtube.com/watch?v=NqR_YkYYw54.

129   Keats, J., Rossetti, W. M., Colvin, S., Shelley, P. B., and Marks, D. (2013). *John Keats completed works ultimate collection 50+ works. All poems, poetry, posthumous works, letters and biography.* First Everlasting Flames Publishing.

MEDITATION: OM AWAY THE BABY BLUES AND SOME OTHER THINGS TOO

131   Puff, R. (July 7, 2013). An overview of meditation: Its origins and traditions. PsychologyToday.com. Retrieved from https://www.psychologytoday.com/blog/meditation-modern-life/201307/overview-meditation-its-origins-and-traditions.

133   Perez-Blasco, J., Viguer, P., and Rodrigo, M. (2013). Effects of a mindfulness-based intervention on psychological distress, well-being, and maternal self-efficacy in breast-feeding mothers: Results of

a pilot study. *Archives of Women's Mental Health,* 16(3), 227–236. doi:10.1007/s00737-013-0337

133   Vieten, C., and Astin, J. (2008). Effects of a mindfulness-based intervention during pregnancy on prenatal stress and mood: results of a pilot study. *Archives of Women's Mental Health,* 11(67), 67–74. doi:10.1007/s00737-008-0214-3

134   Dimidjian, S., Goodman, S. H., Felder, J. N., Gallop, R., Brown, A. P., and Beck, A. (2016). Staying well during pregnancy and the postpartum: A pilot randomized trial of mindfulness-based cognitive therapy for the prevention of depressive relapse/recurrence. *Journal of Consulting and Clinical Psychology,* 84(2), 134–45. doi:10.1037/ccp0000068

135   Gambrel, L. E., and Piercy, F. P. (2015). Mindfulness-based relationship education for couples expecting their first child—part 2: Phenomenological findings. *Journal of Marital & Family Therapy,* 41(1), 25–41. doi:10.1111/jmft.12065

136   Naumberg, C. (May 2, 2015). Mindfulness: the definition (part 1 of 6). *Mindful Parenting* (blog). *PsychCentral.* Retrieved from https://blogs.psych central.com/mindful-parenting/2015/05/917.

141   Naumberg, C. (September 5, 2015). Meditation for parents: The 20-minute activity we all should try. HuffingtonPost.com. Retrieved from http://www .huffingtonpost.com/2013/09/05/meditation-for -parents-mindful-parenting-carla-naumburg_n _3870108.html?utm_hp_ref=stress-less-parenting.

141   Vieten, C. (2009). *Mindful Motherhood*. Oakland, CA: New Harbinger Publications.

142   Vieten, C. (January 24, 2011). Mindful awareness of breathing meditation. Audio recording. Retrieved from https://s3.amazonaws.com/ions-assets/library /audio/MindfulAwarenessOfBreathingMeditation .mp3.

143   Ibid.

AND BABY MAKES THREE: HOW BRINGING BABY HOME CAN BRING A COUPLE CLOSER TOGETHER

147   Senior, J. (2014). *All Joy and No Fun*. New York, NY: Ecco.

153   Ehrenfeld, T. (October 15, 2013). 36 questions to bring you closer together. Web blog post. Retrieved from https://www.psychologytoday.com/blog/open -gently/201310/36-questions-bring-you-closer -together.

TALK IS *NOT* CHEAP: THE VALUE OF TALK THERAPY

169   Foa, E. B. (2010). Cognitive behavioral therapy of obsessive-compulsive disorder. *Dialogues in Clinical Neuroscience, 12*(2), 199–207.

170   Mureşan Madar, and Băban. (2015). The development and piloting of a CBT group program for

postpartum depression. *Journal of Evidence-Based Psychotherapies, 15*(1), 51–64.

170   EMDR International Association. How does EMDR work. Retrieved from http://www.emdria.org/general /custom.asp?page=119.

ABOUT THE AUTHOR

Dayna M. Kurtz, LMSW, CPT, is a leading authority on the subject of mothercare and serves as director of the Anna Keefe Women's Center at the Training Institute for Mental Health in Manhattan. She is a licensed social worker and NASM (National Academy of Sports Medicine) Certified Personal Trainer with an additional certification in training pre- and postnatal clients. Dayna is the author of *The Female Body Fix* and is a contributor to *The Doctors Book of Home Remedies* (both published by Rodale). Dayna serves as a Real Answers expert on TheBump.com. She has written or been consulted on articles for the websites of *The Today Show, Pregnancy & Newborn, Popsugar, Big City Moms, Pregnancy Corner,* and *WAGmagazine* among others, and writes the *Mother Matters* blog for the *Huffington Post*. A sought-after speaker, Dayna regularly presents on the subject of women transitioning to motherhood. She lives in New York City with her family.

ABOUT FAMILIUS

VISIT OUR WEBSITE: WWW.FAMILIUS.COM

JOIN OUR FAMILY

There are lots of ways to connect with us! Subscribe to our news-letters at www.familius.com to receive uplifting daily inspiration, essays from our Pater Familius, a free ebook every month, and the first word on special discounts and Familius news.

GET BULK DISCOUNTS

If you feel a few friends and family might benefit from what you've read, let us know and we'll be happy to provide you with quantity discounts. Simply email us at orders@familius.com.

CONNECT

- Facebook: www.facebook.com/paterfamilius
- Twitter: @familiustalk, @paterfamilius1
- Pinterest: www.pinterest.com/familius
- Instagram: @familiustalk

FAMILIUS

The most important work you ever do will be within the walls of your own home.

CPSIA information can be obtained
at www.ICGtesting.com
Printed in the USA
FSOW01n1353030318
45195FS